THE
40 MOST BEAUTIFUL
CLASSIC CARS
IN THE WORLD

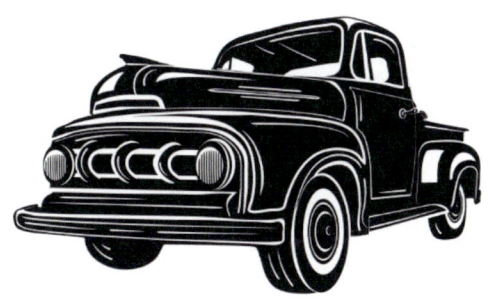

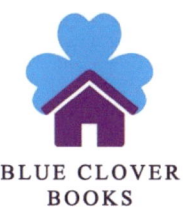

BLUE CLOVER
BOOKS

Copyright © 2022 Blue Clover Books

All Rights Reserved.

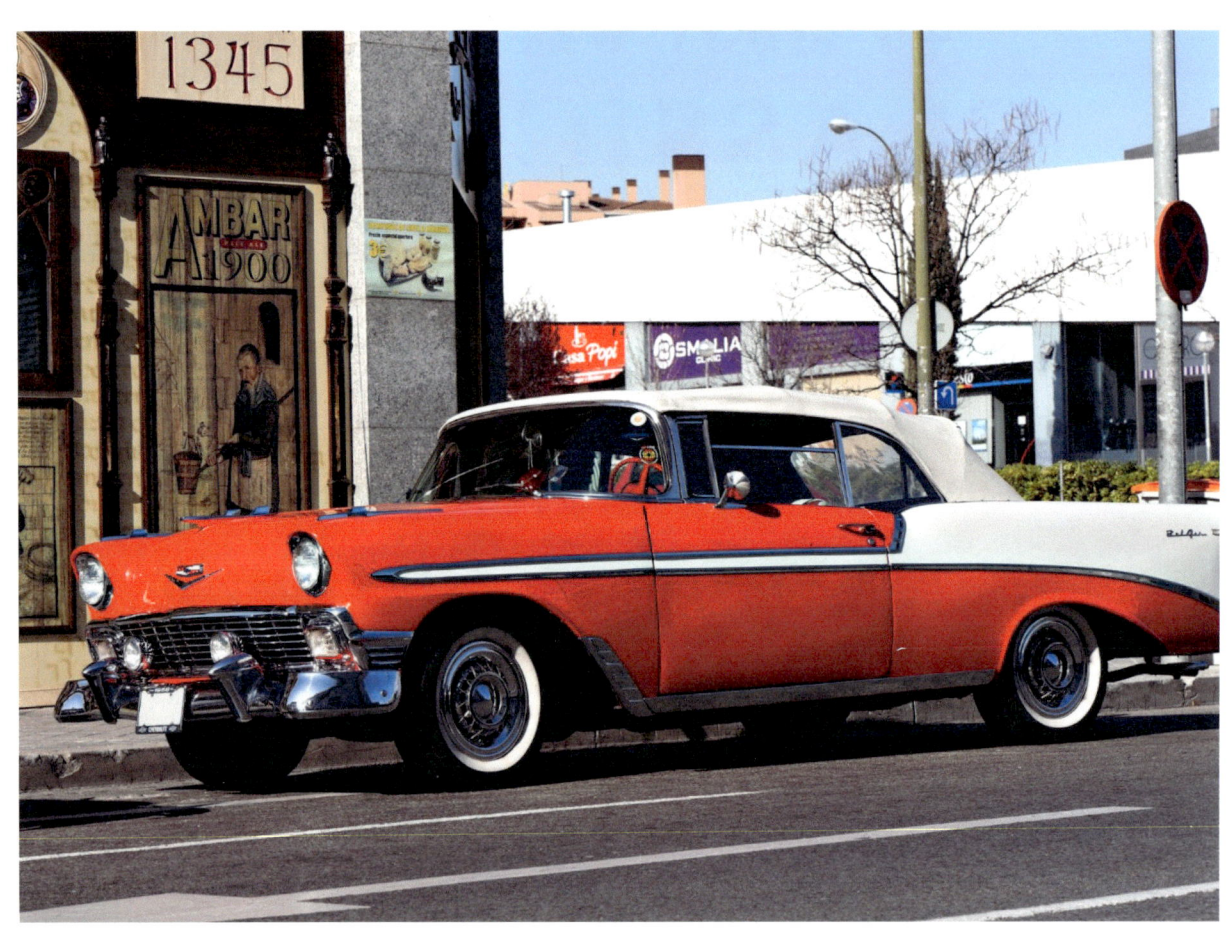

1955 CHEVY BEL AIR

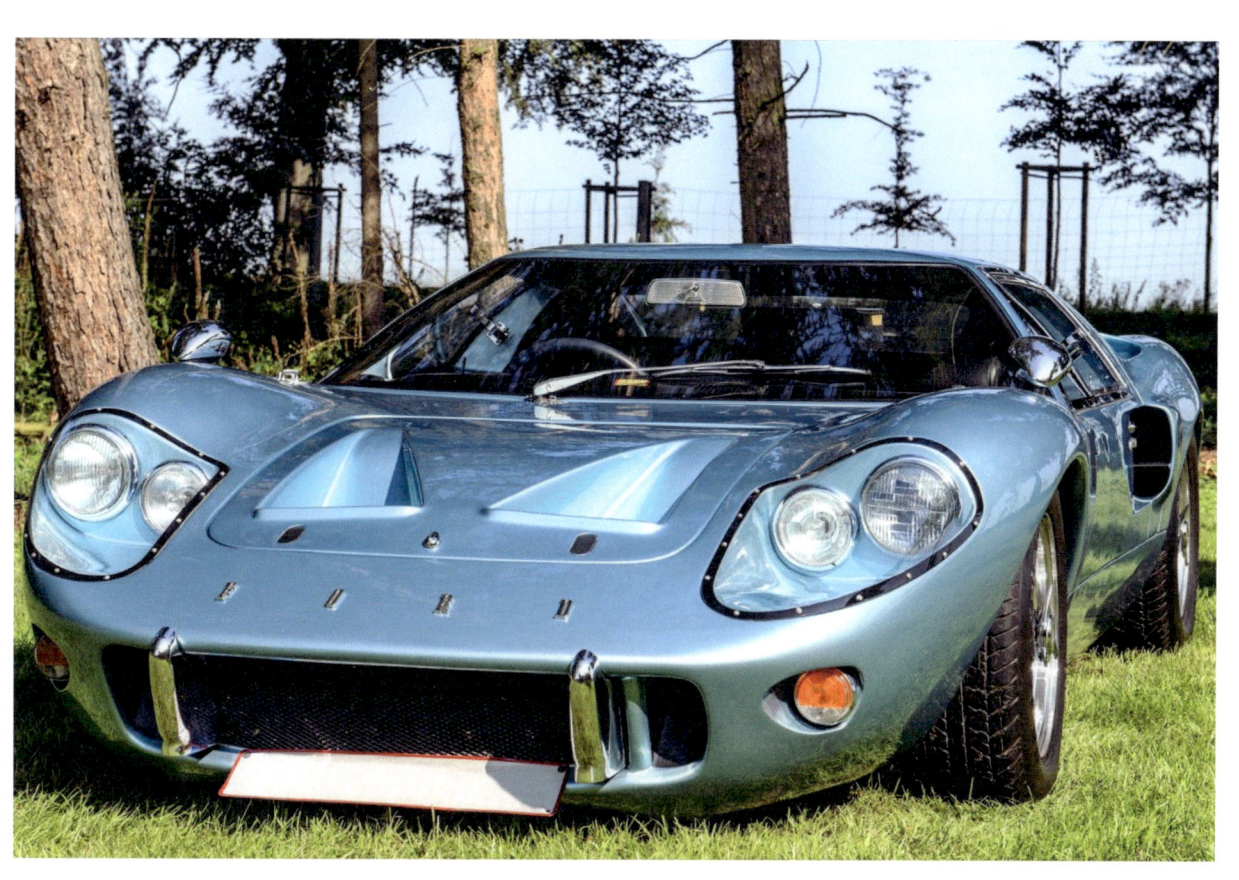

FORD GT40

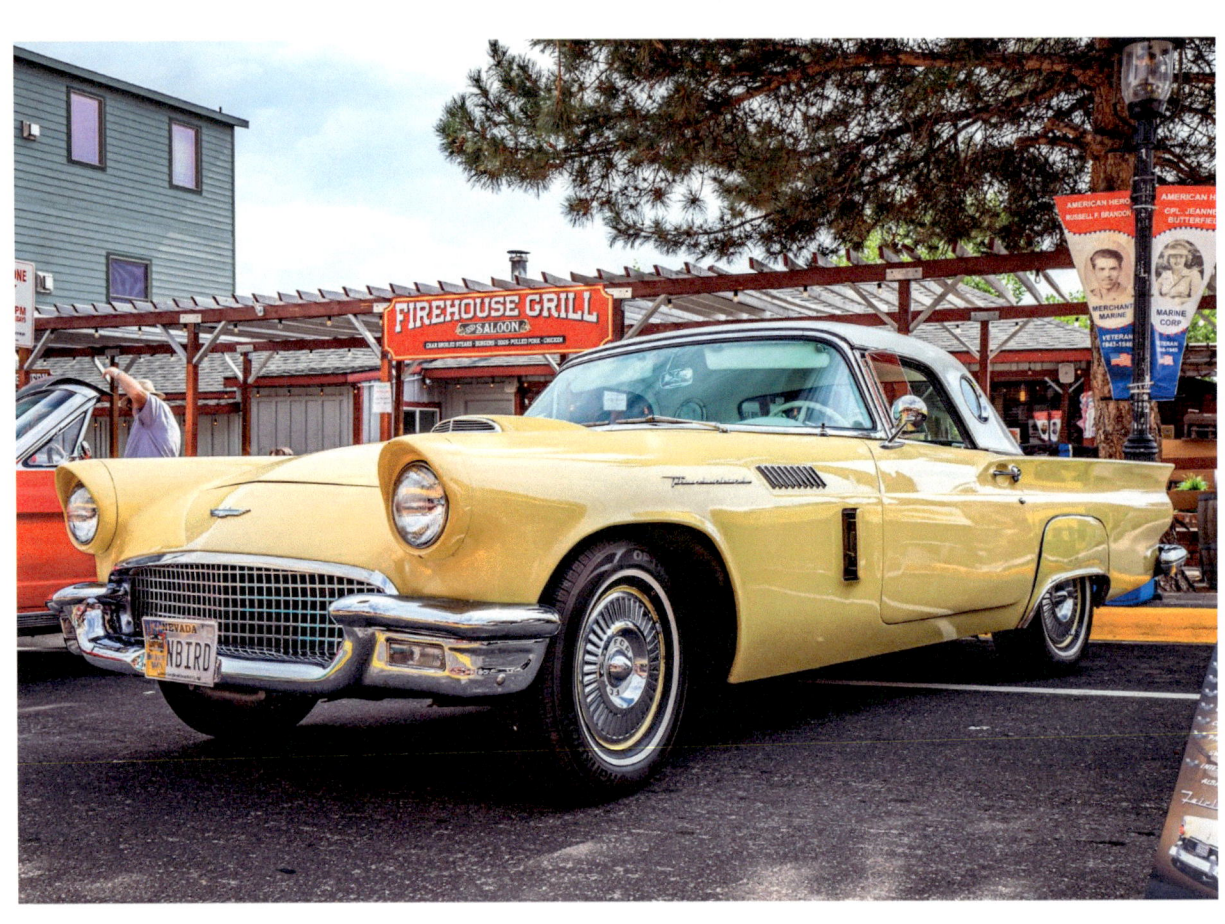

1957 FORD THUNDERBIRD

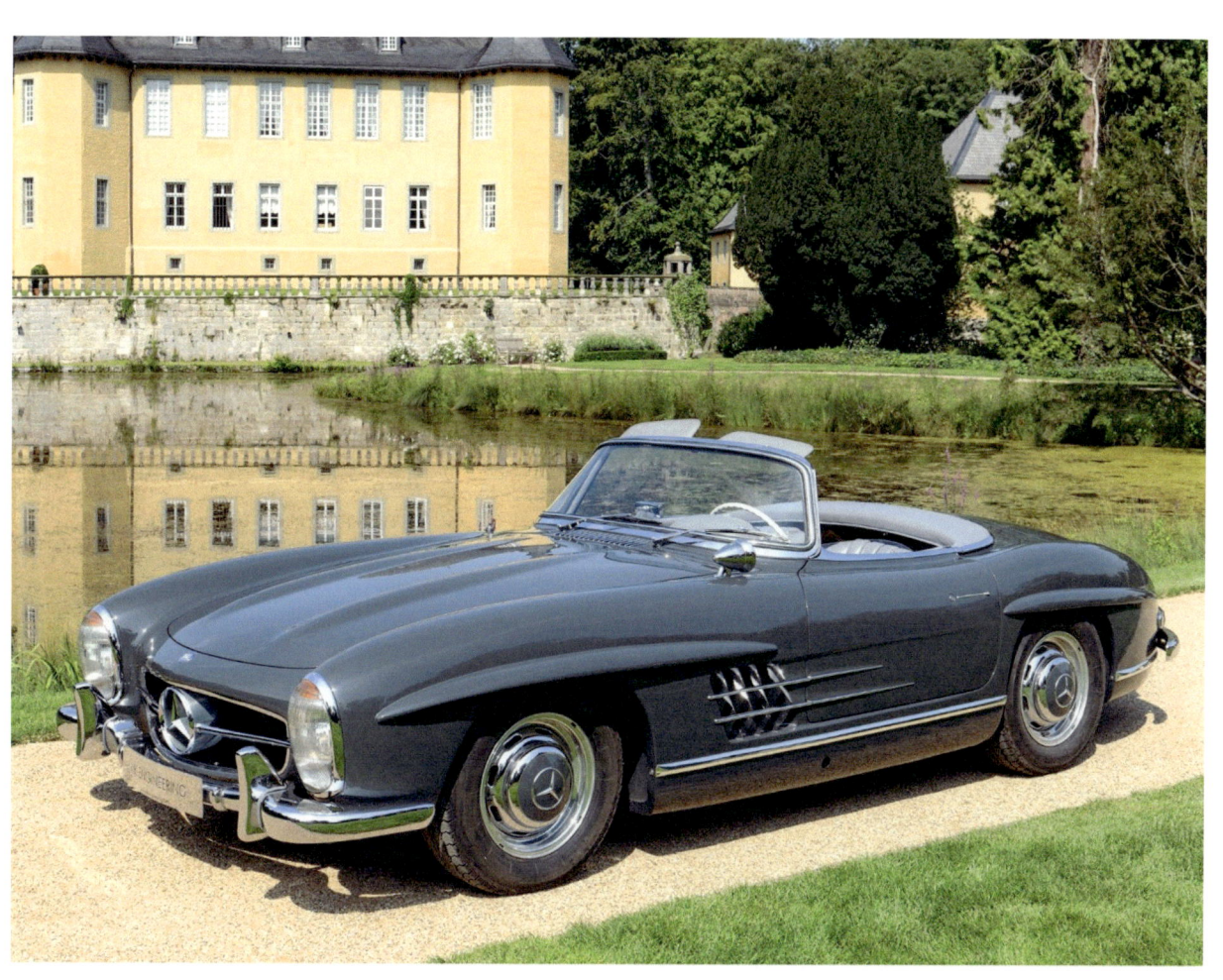

MERCEDES BENZ 300SL

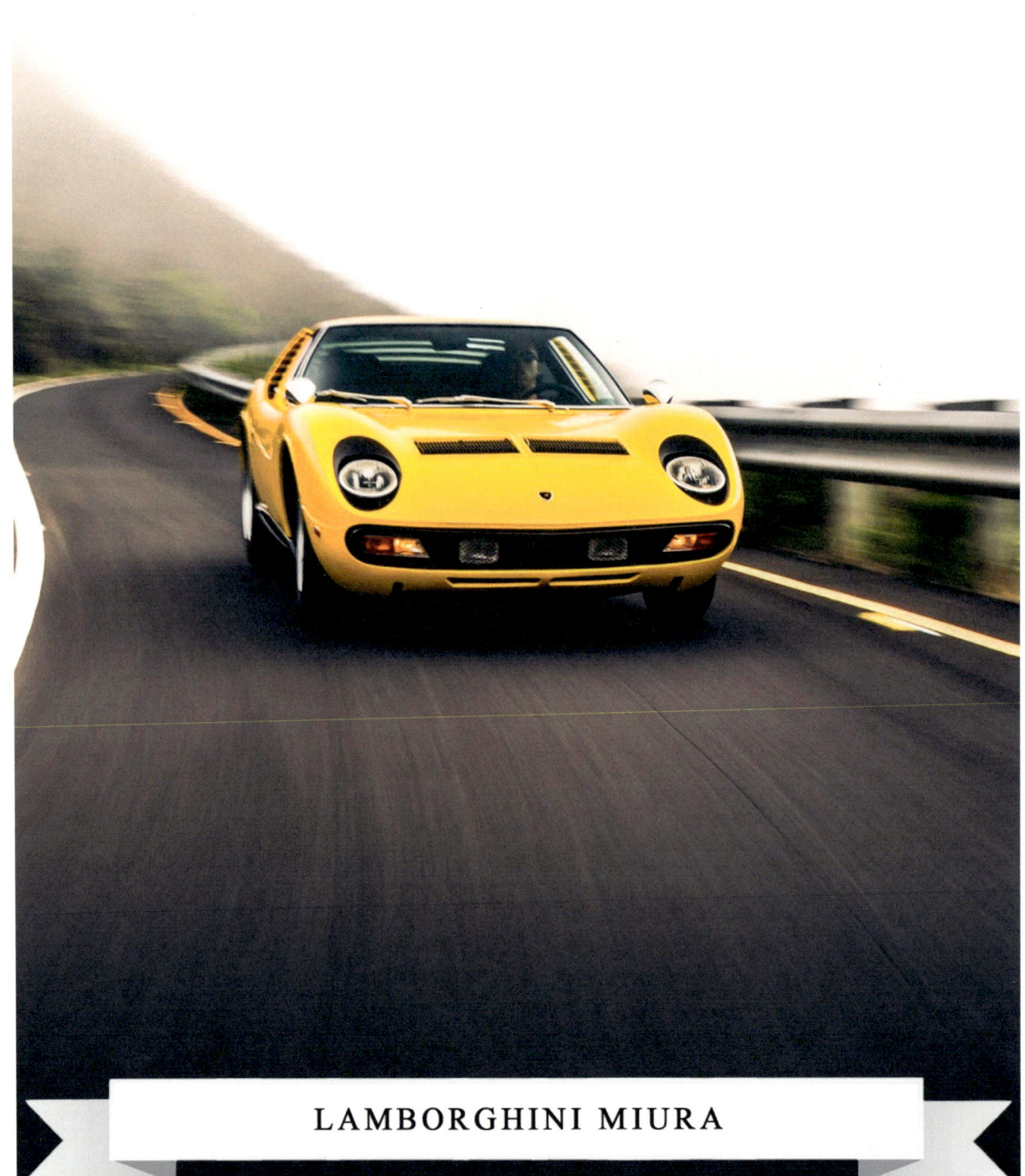

LAMBORGHINI MIURA

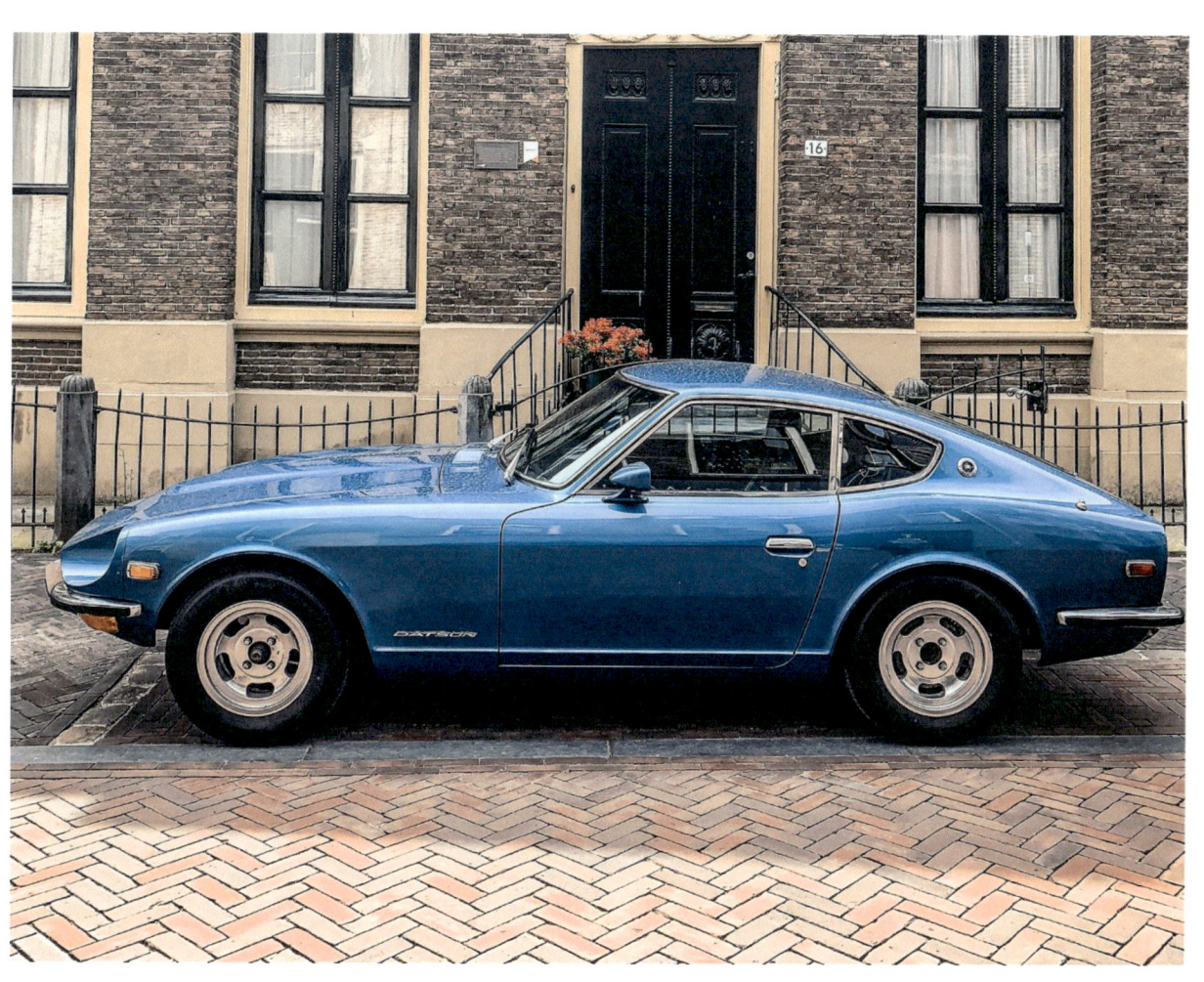

DATSUN 240Z

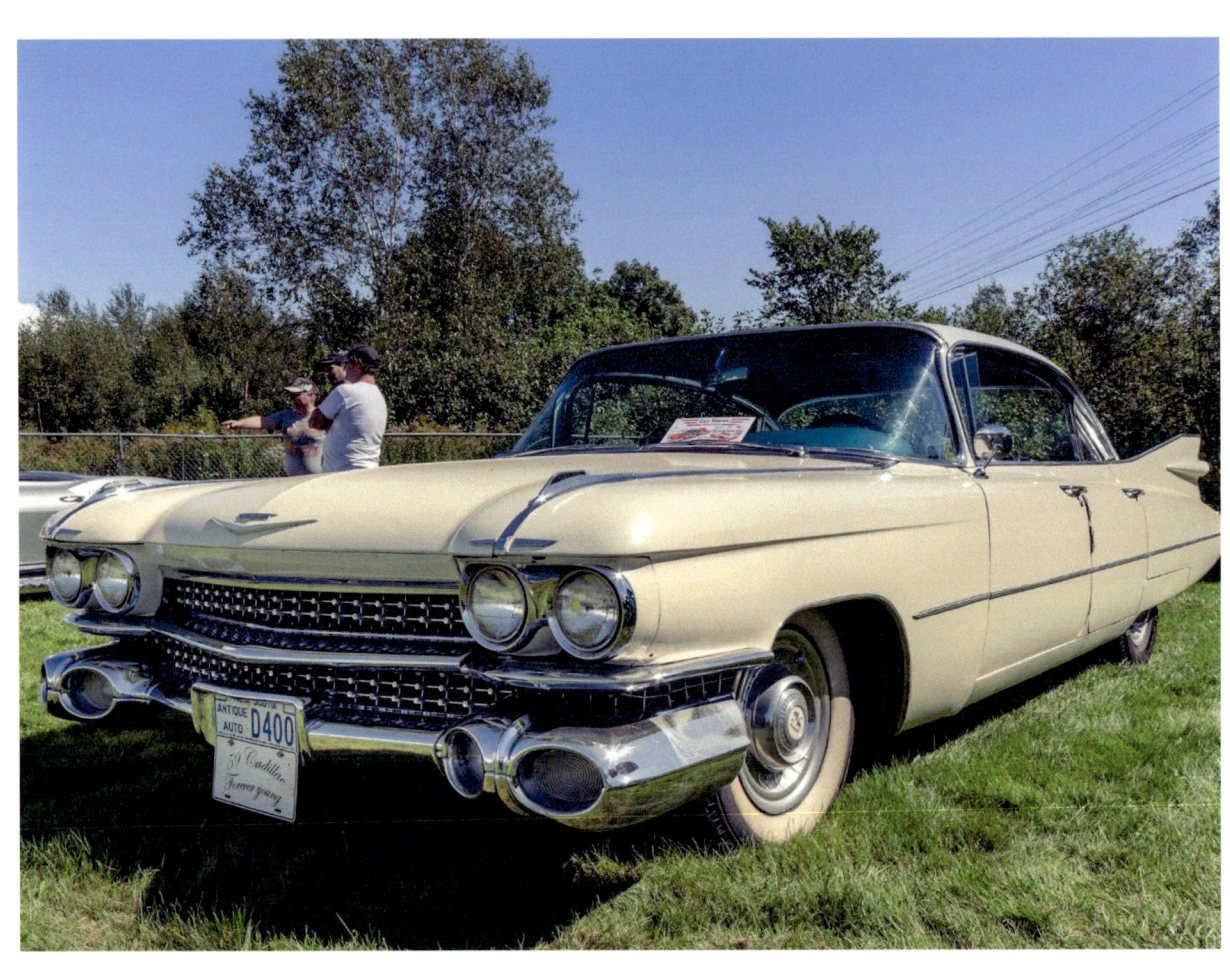

1959 CADILLAC ELDORADO

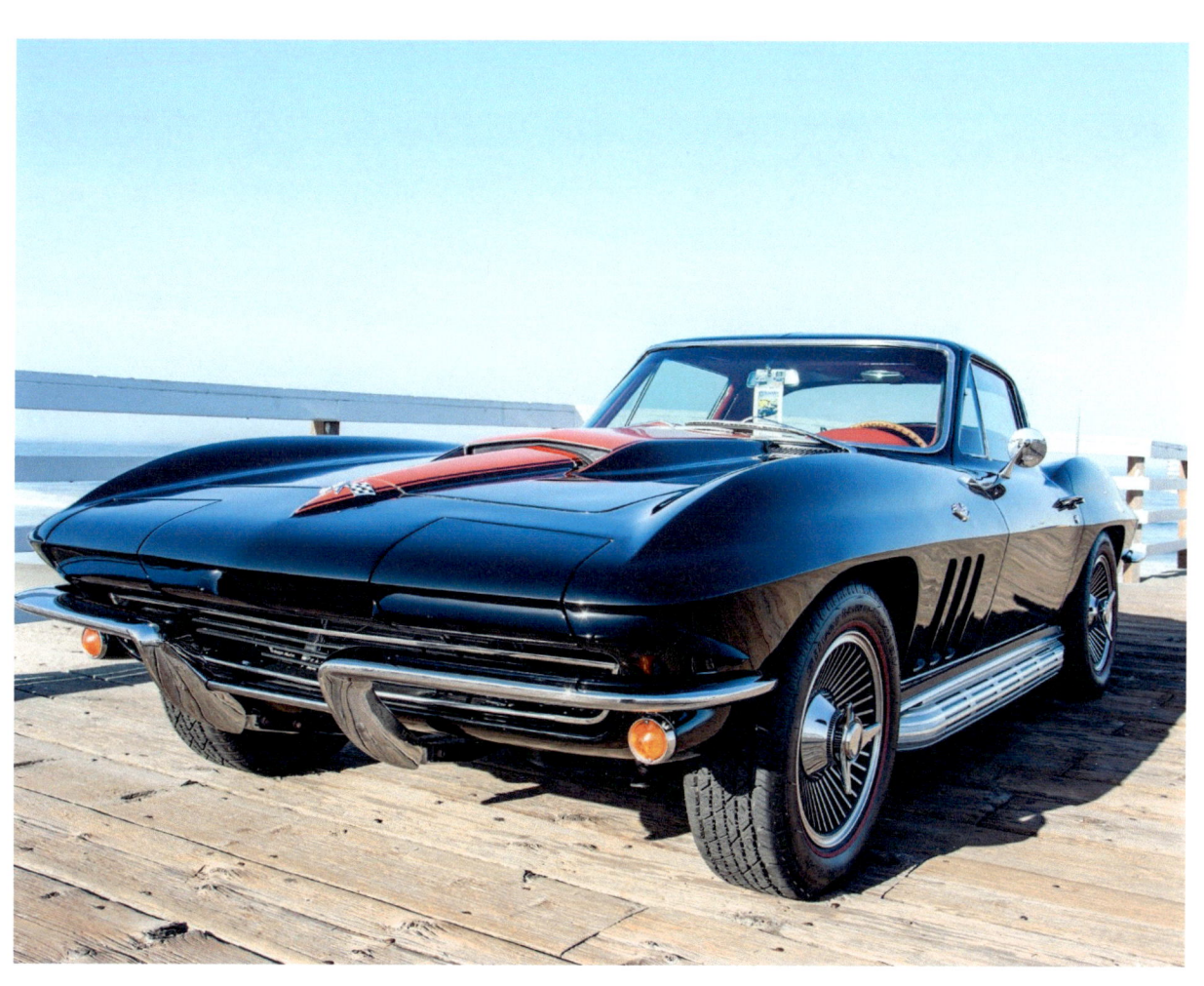

1967 CORVETTE

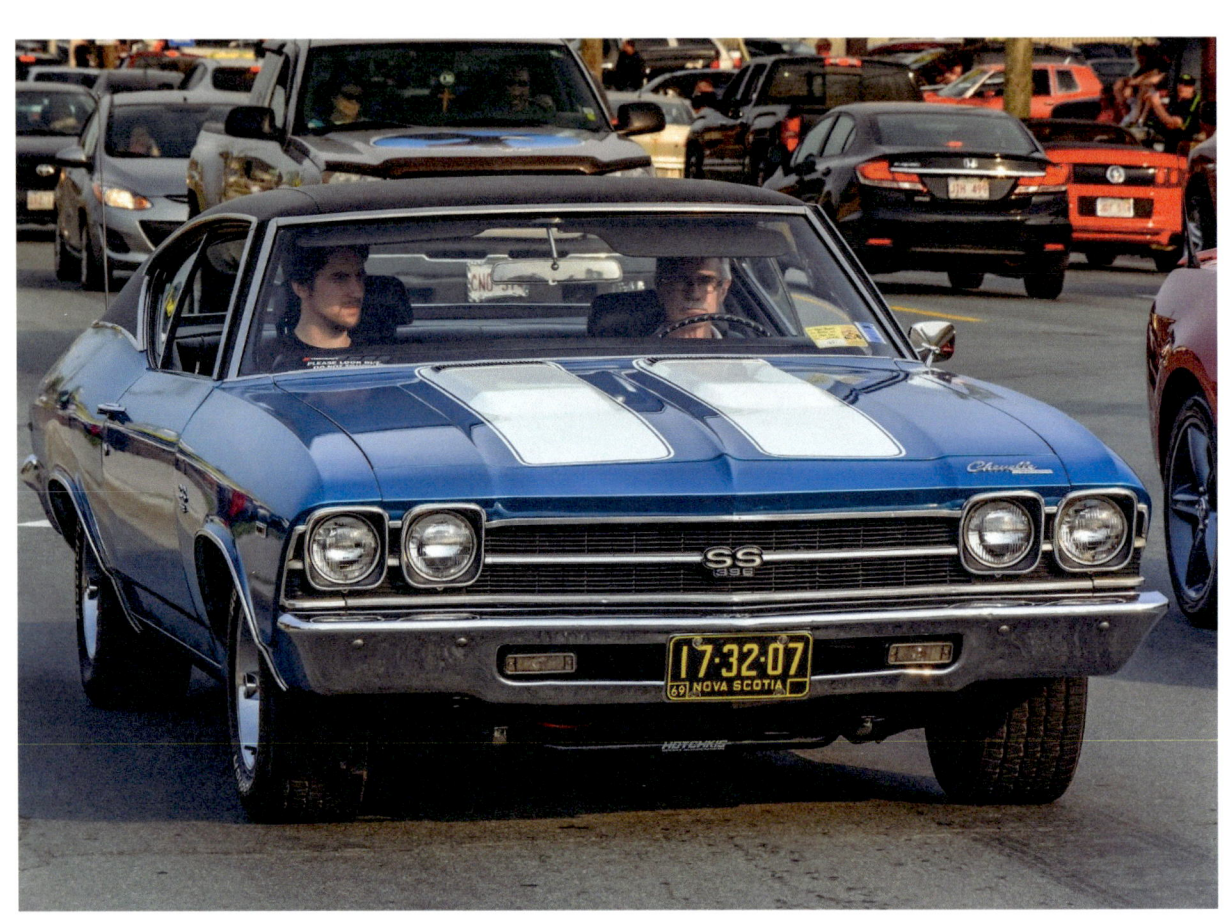

1969 CHEVELLE

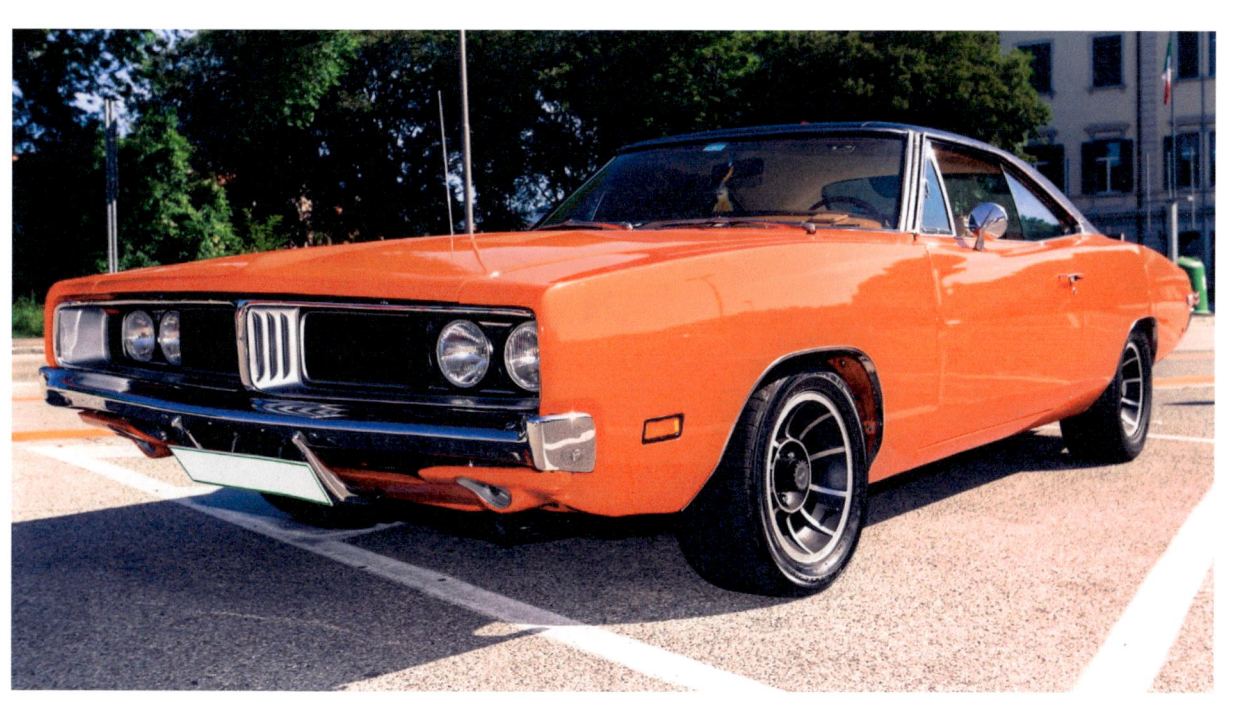

1969 DODGE CHARGER

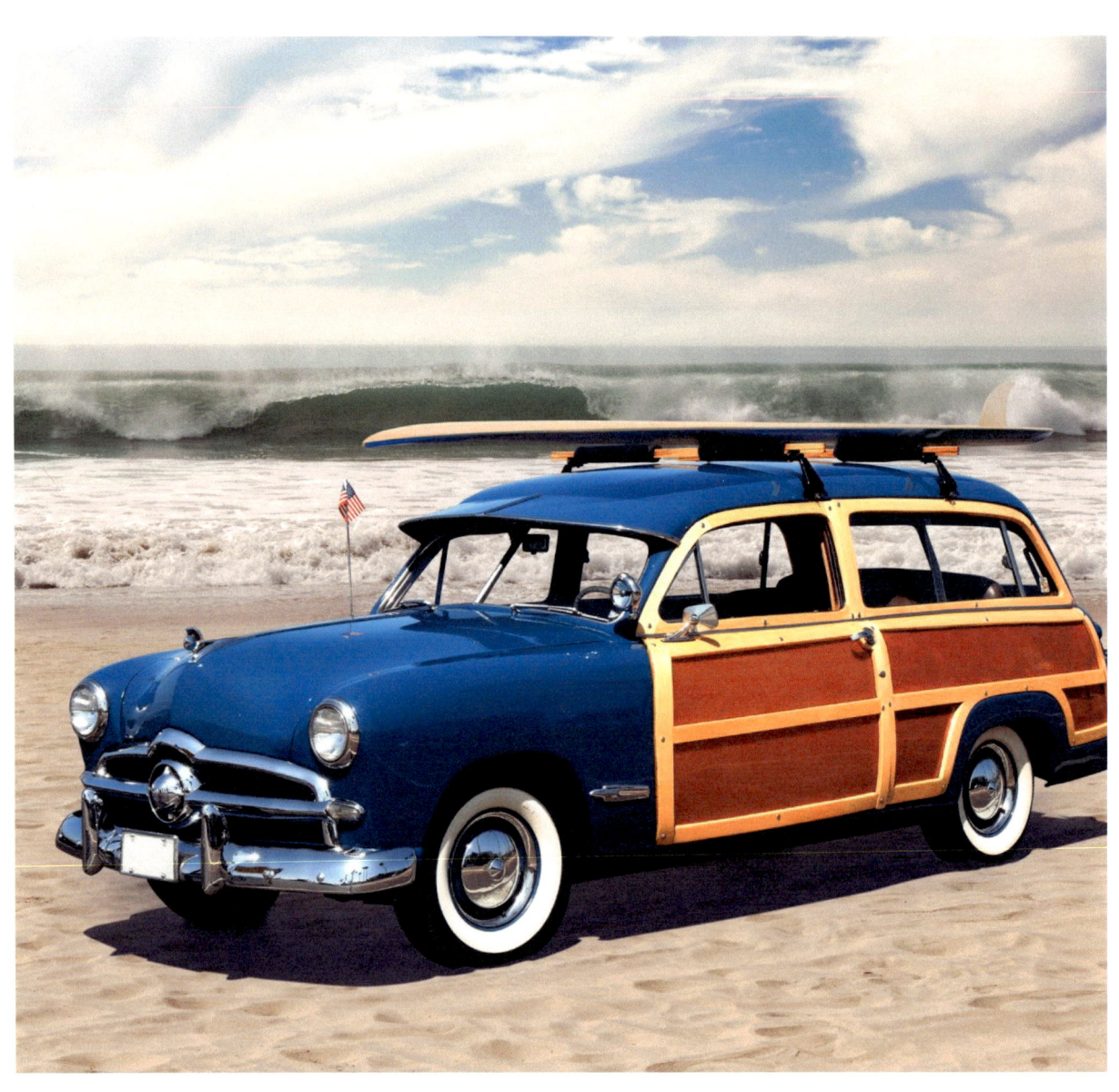

WOODIE

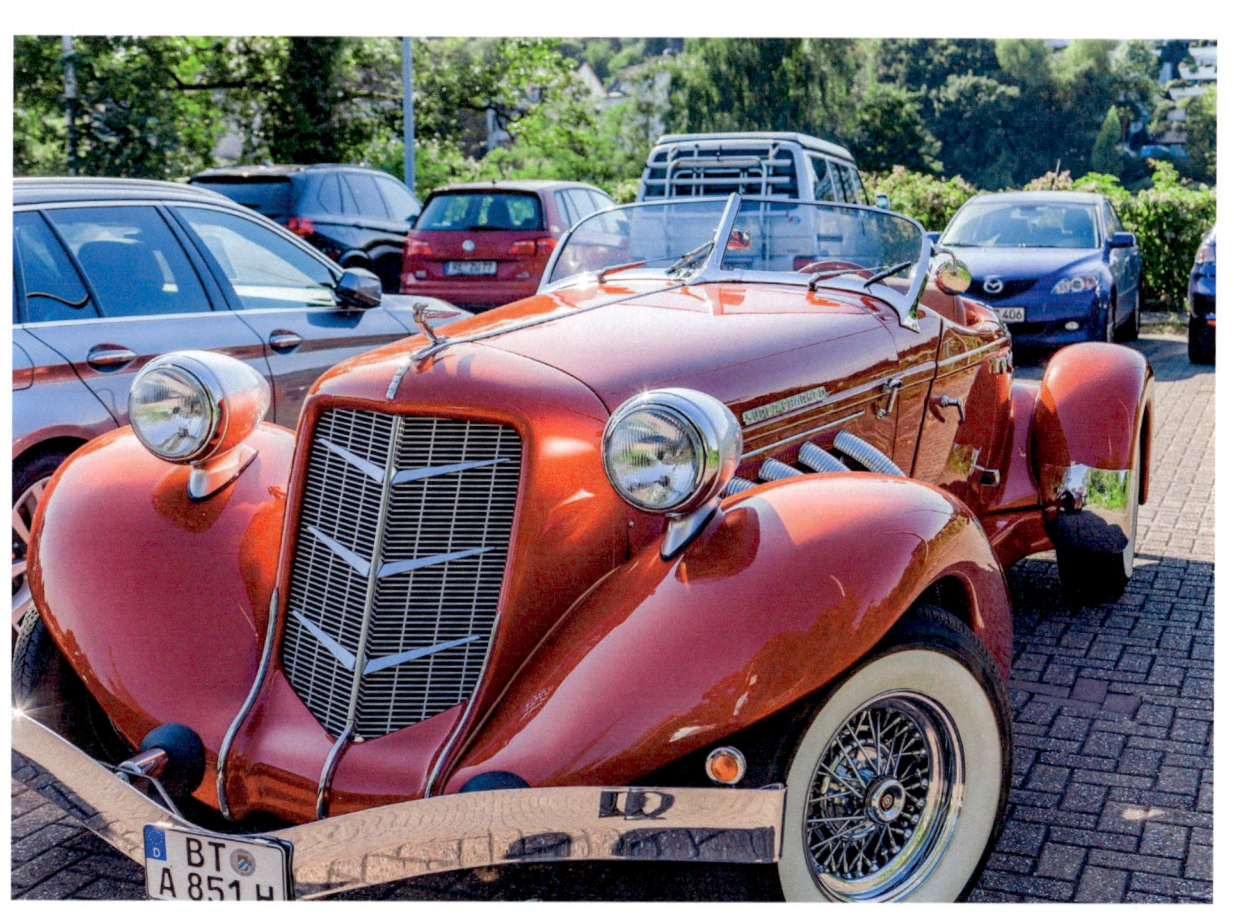

851 BOATTAIL CLASSIC

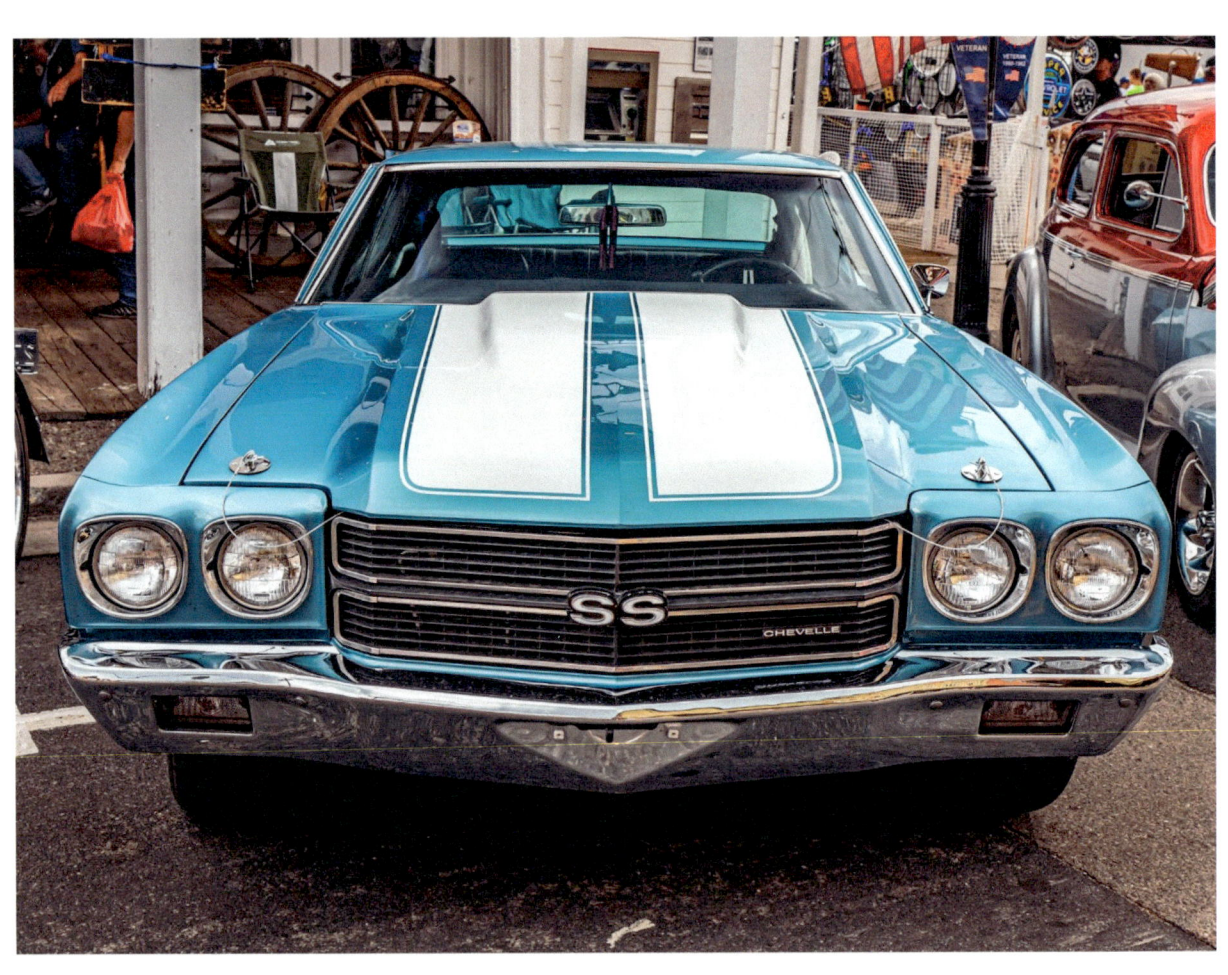

1970 CHEVROLET MALIBU

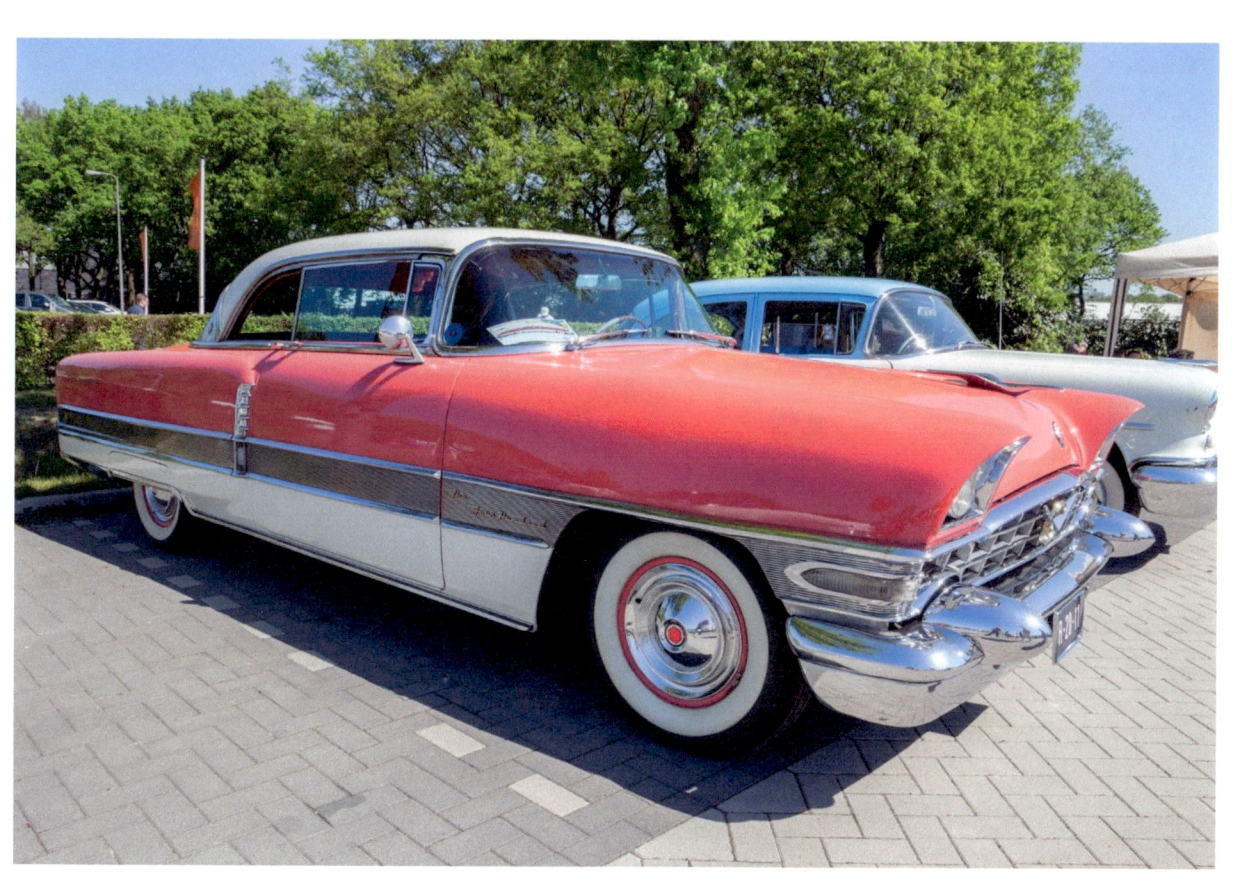

1956 PACKARD FOUR HUNDRED

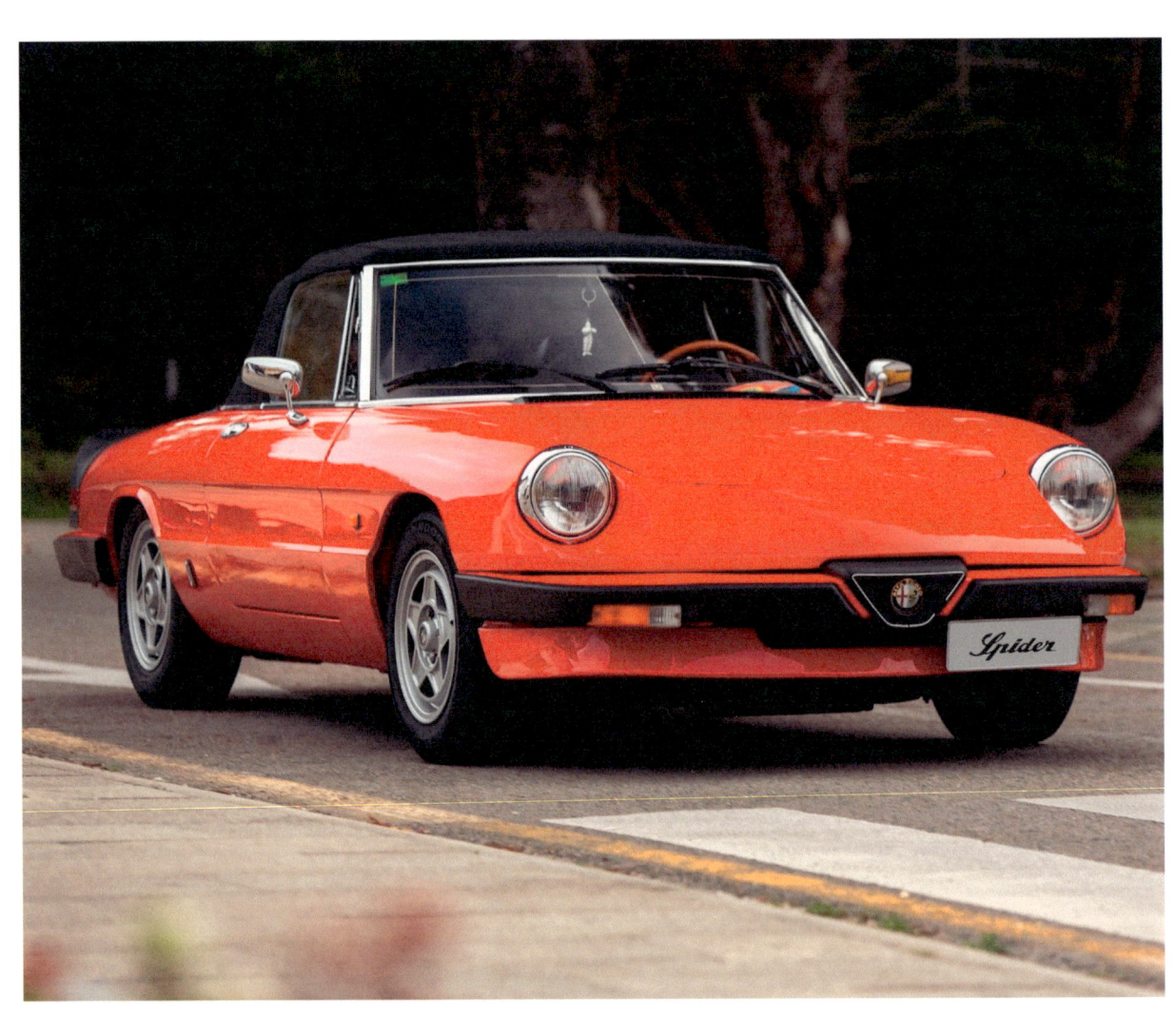

ALFA ROMEO SPIDER

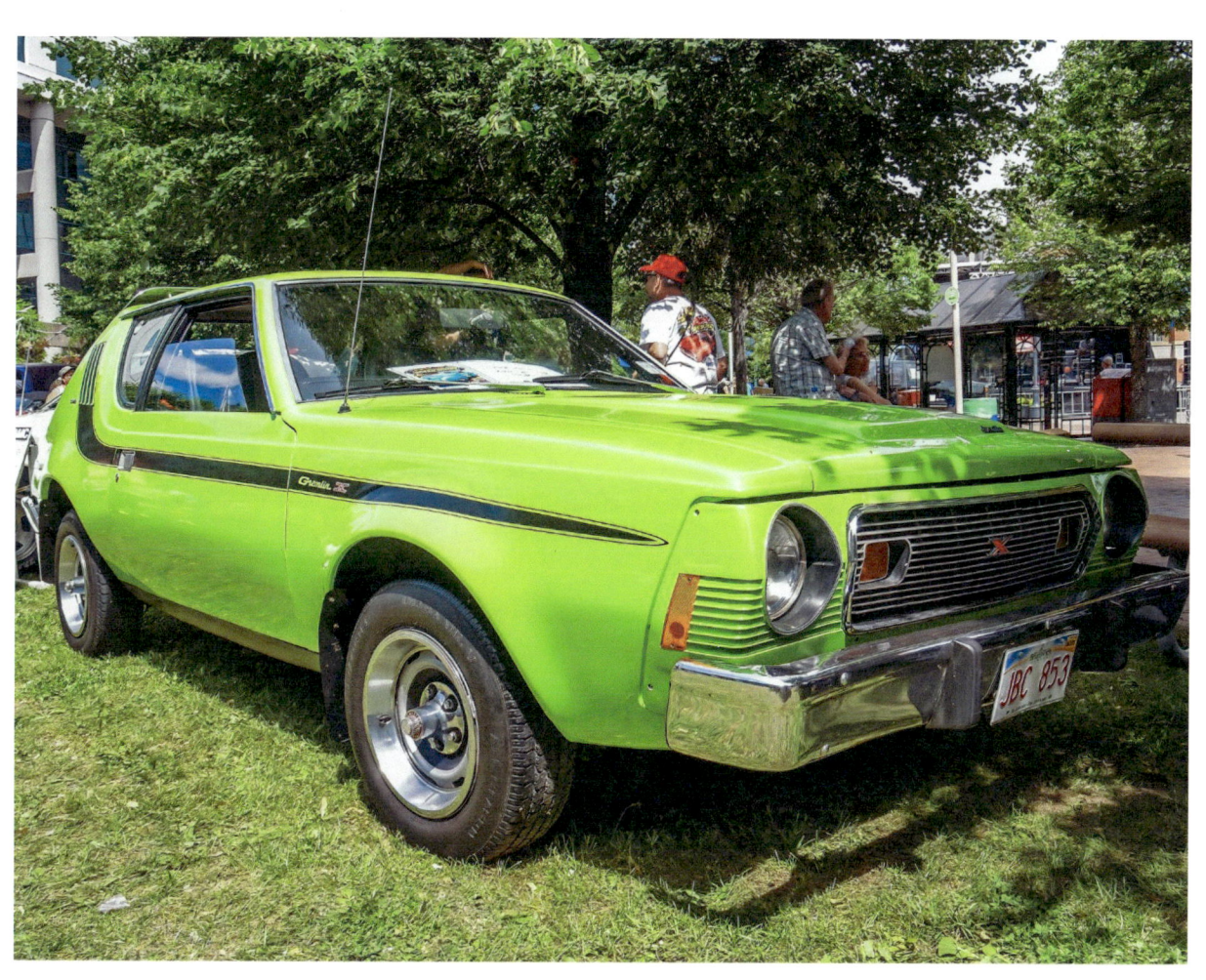

AMC GREMLIN

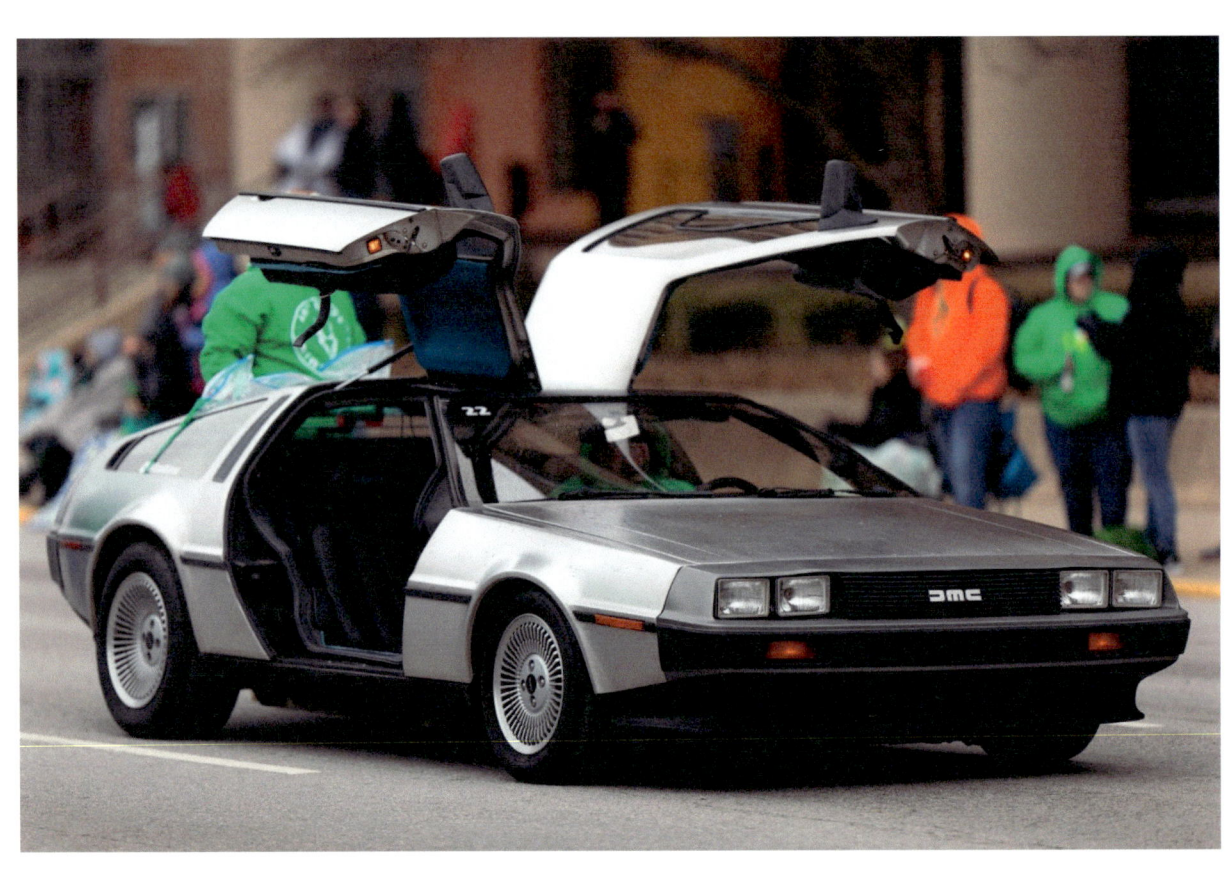

DELOREAN

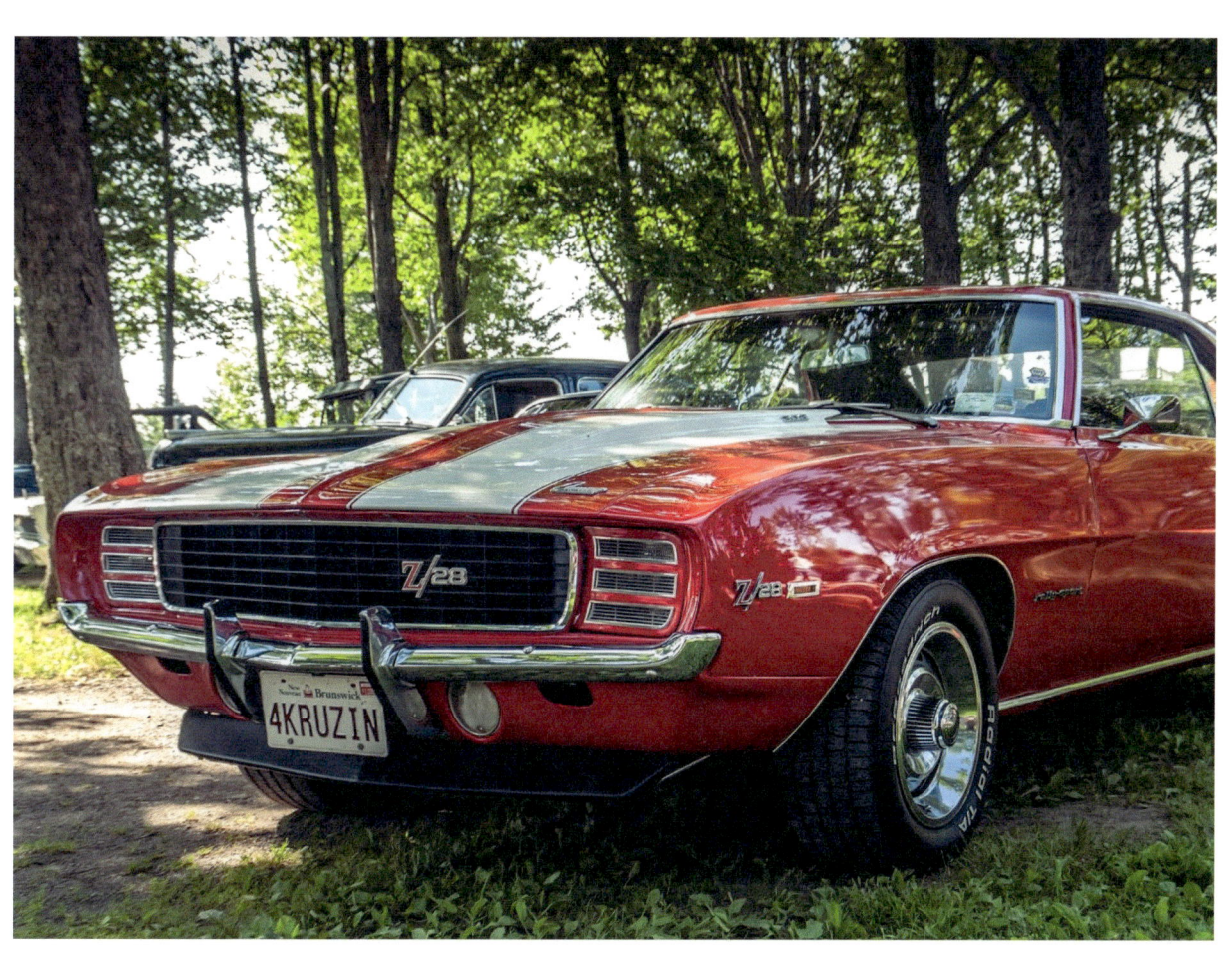

1969 CHEVY CAMARO

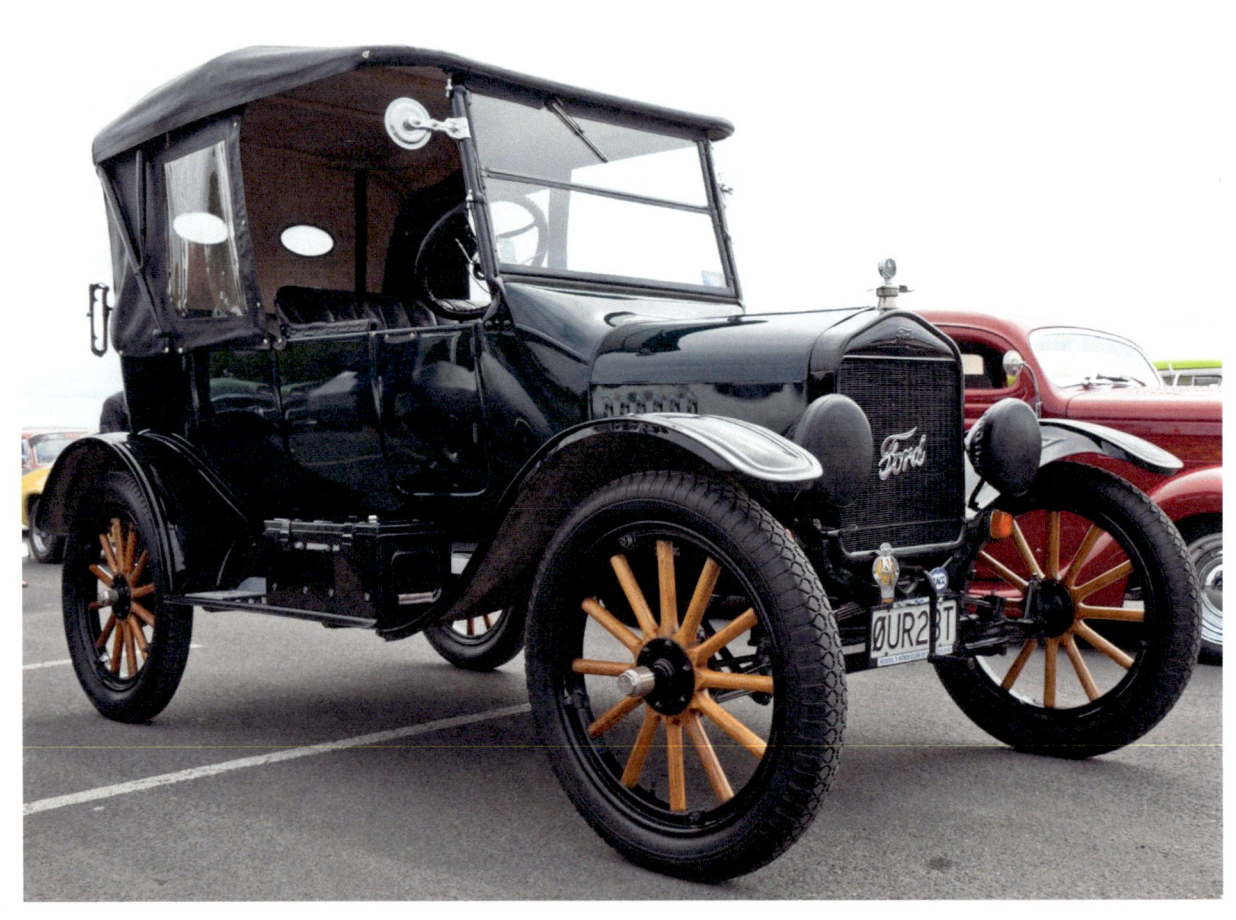

FORD MODEL T

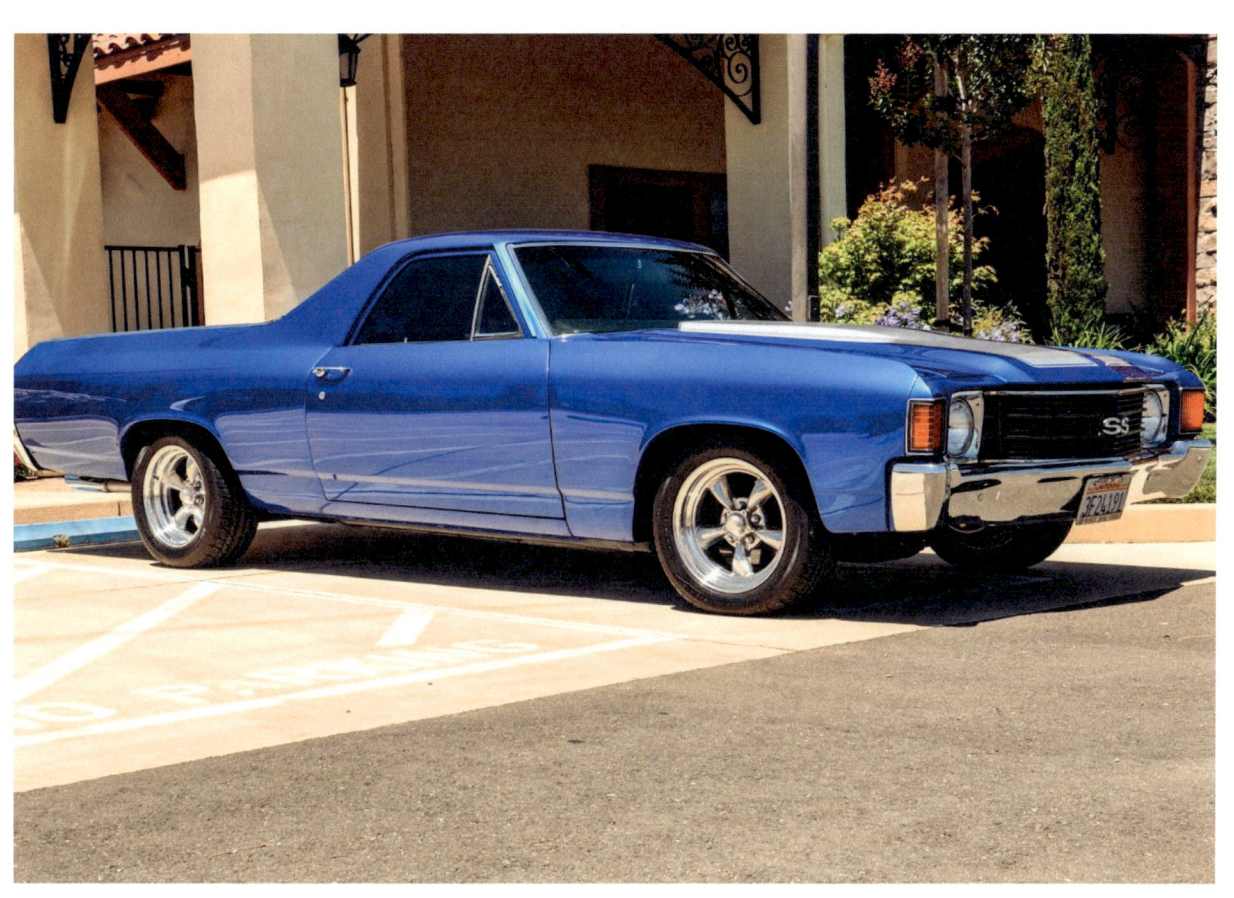

EL CAMINO

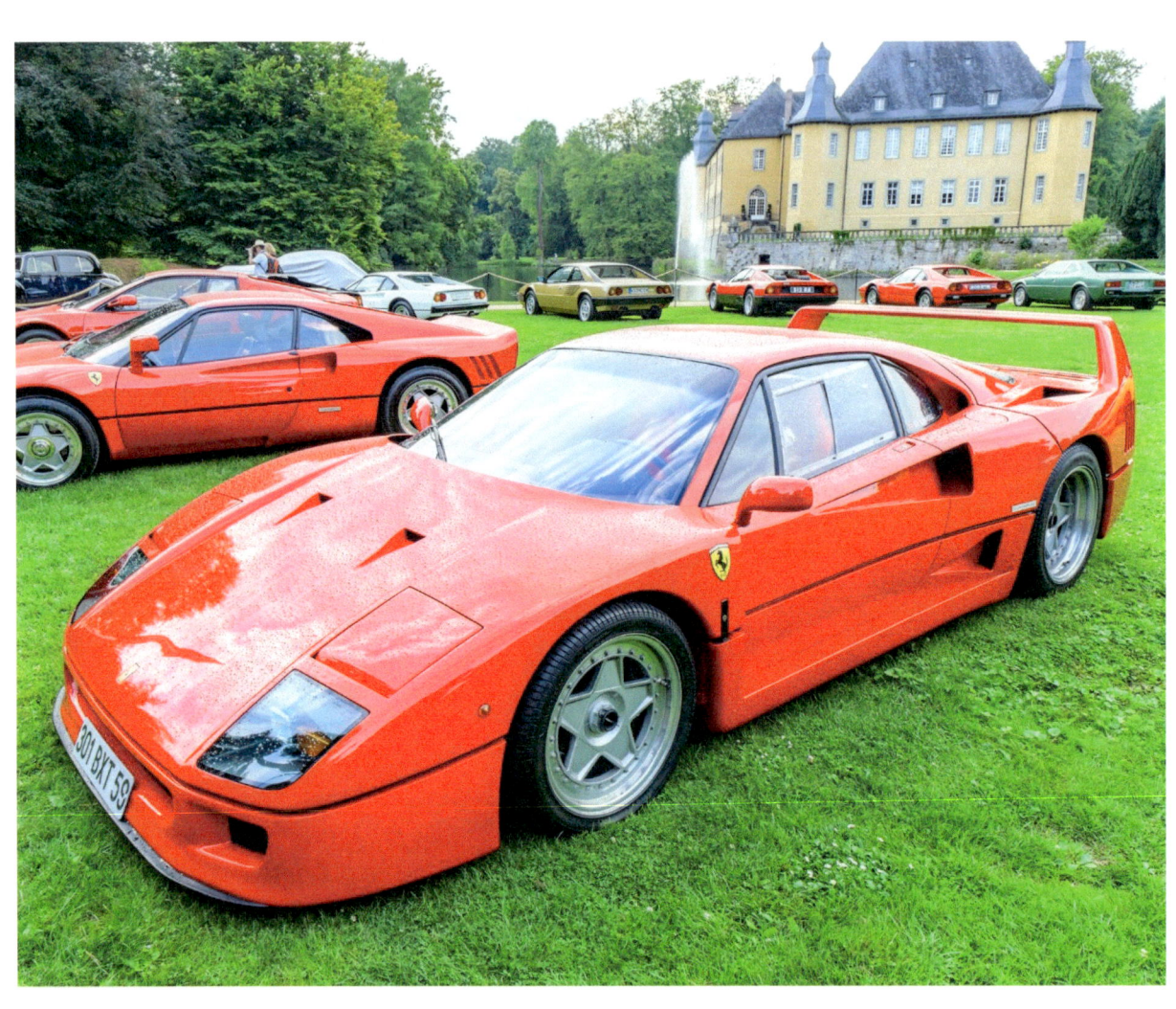

FERRARI 288

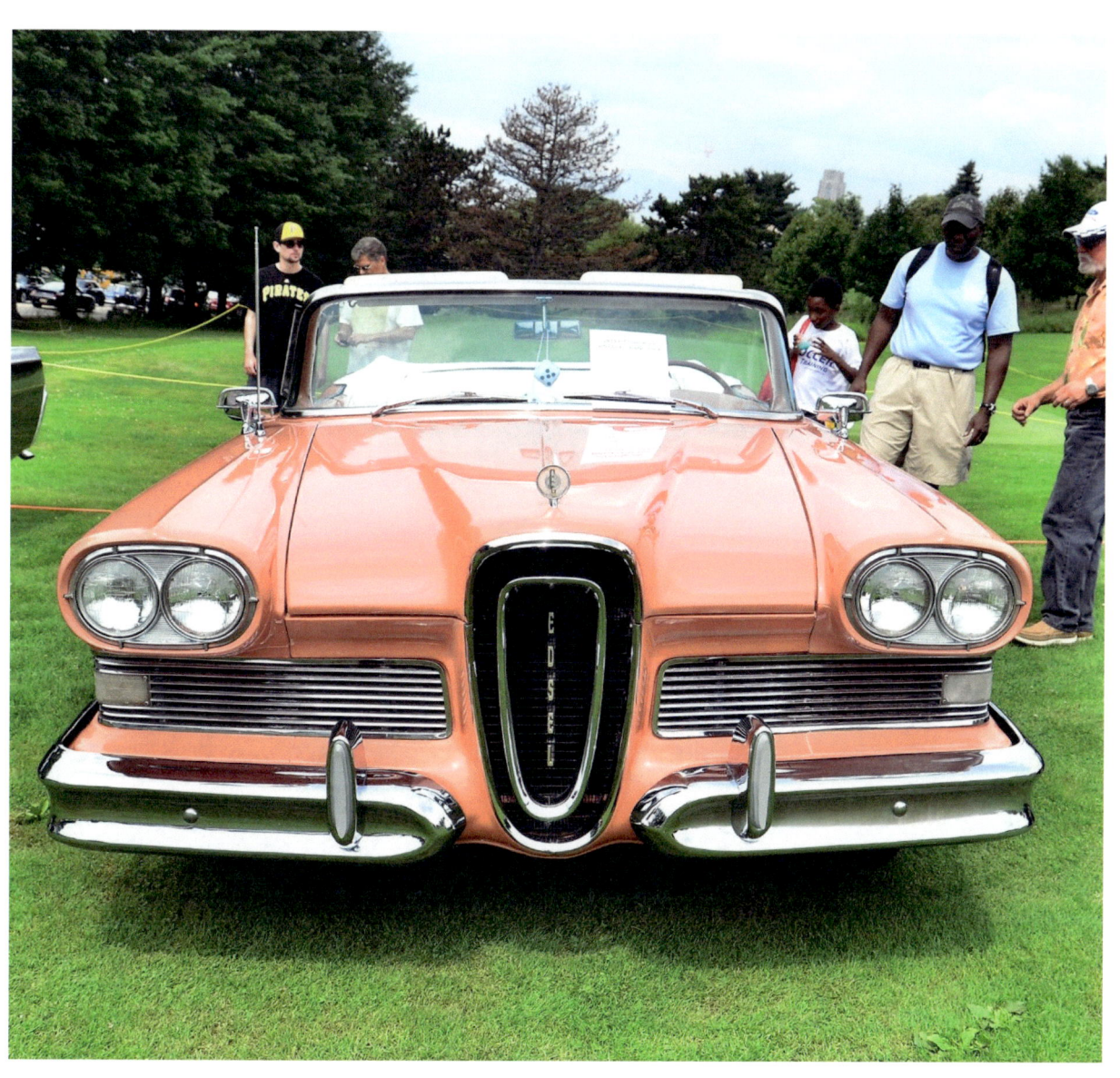

FORD EDSEL

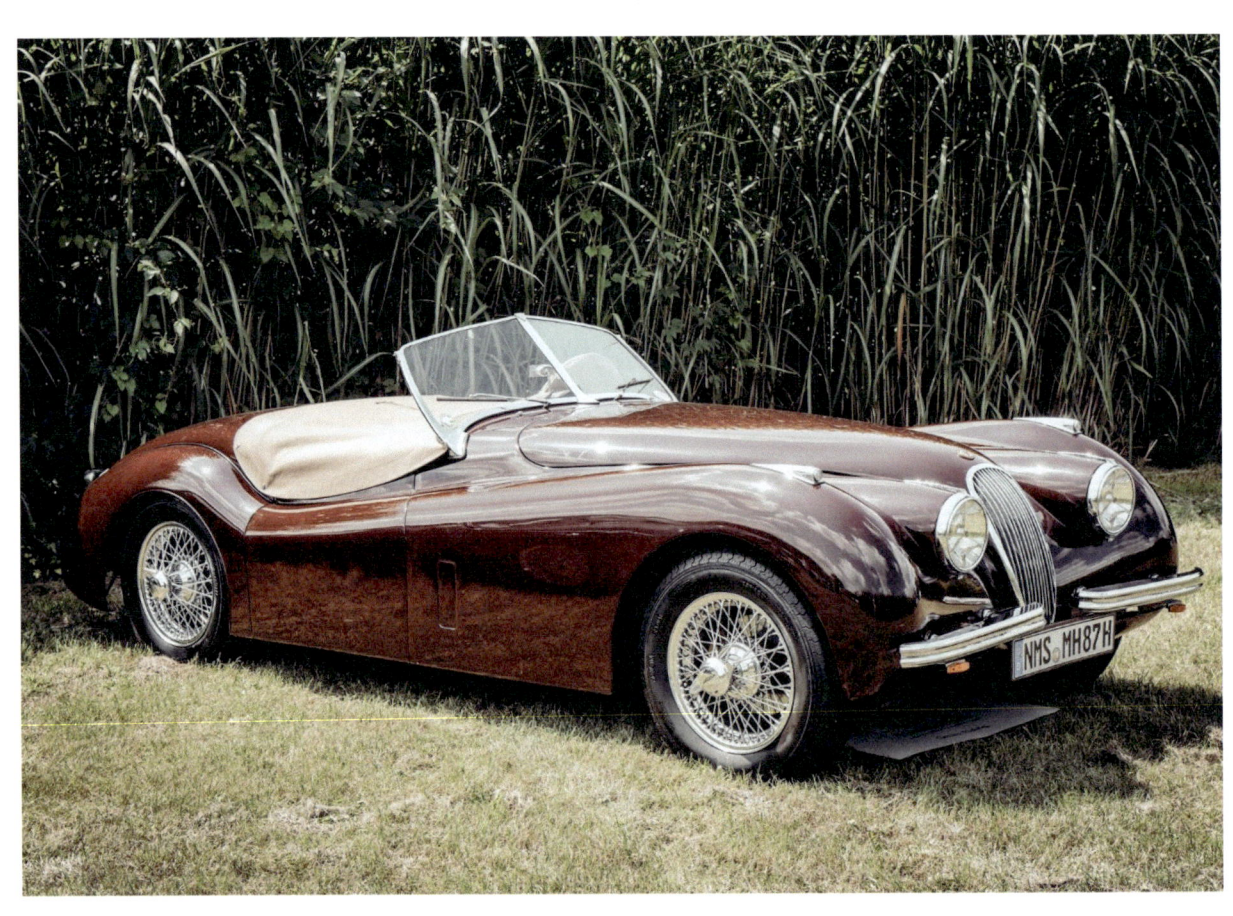

JAGUAR XK120

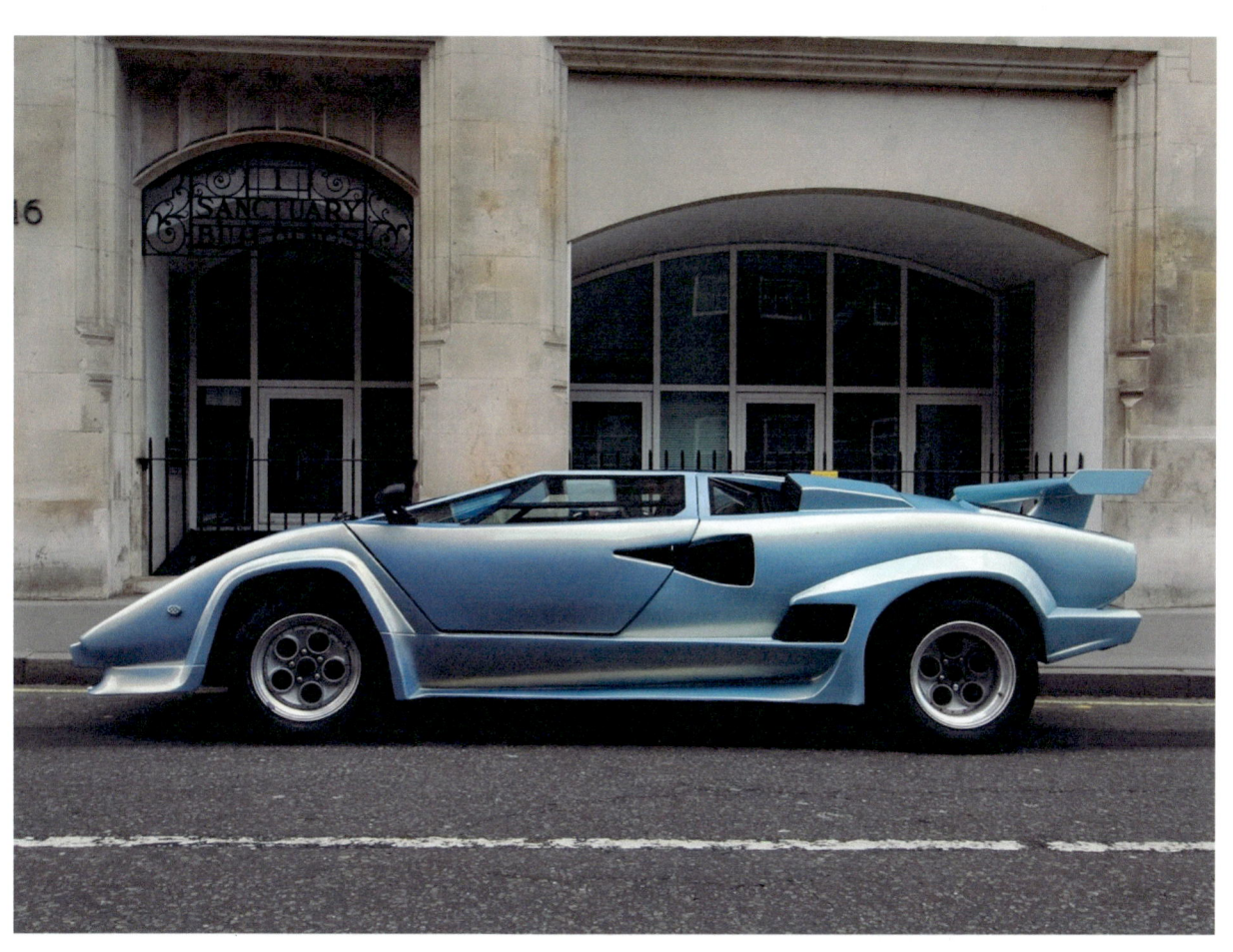

LAMBORGHINI COUNTACH

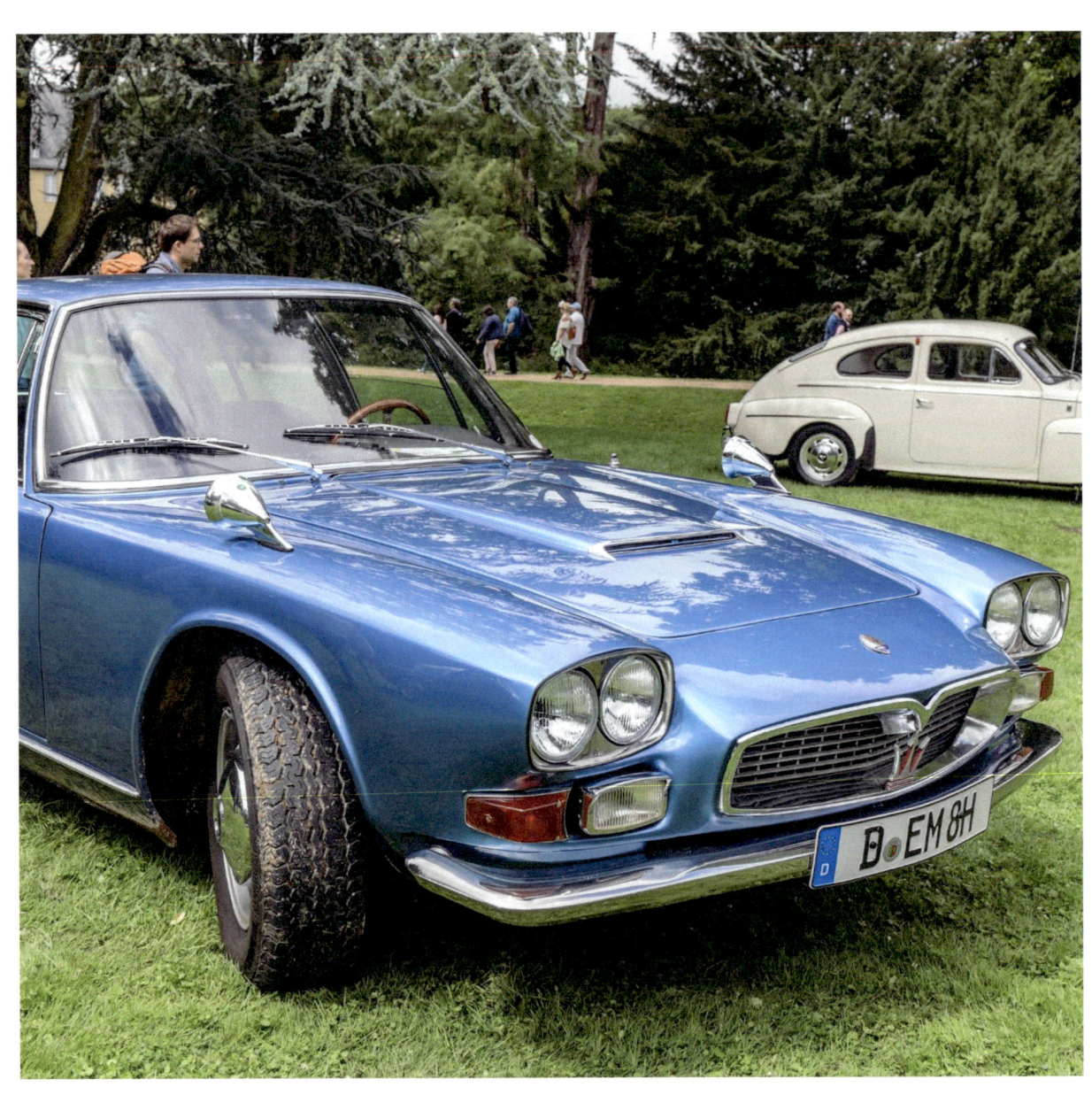

MASERATI QUATTROPORTE

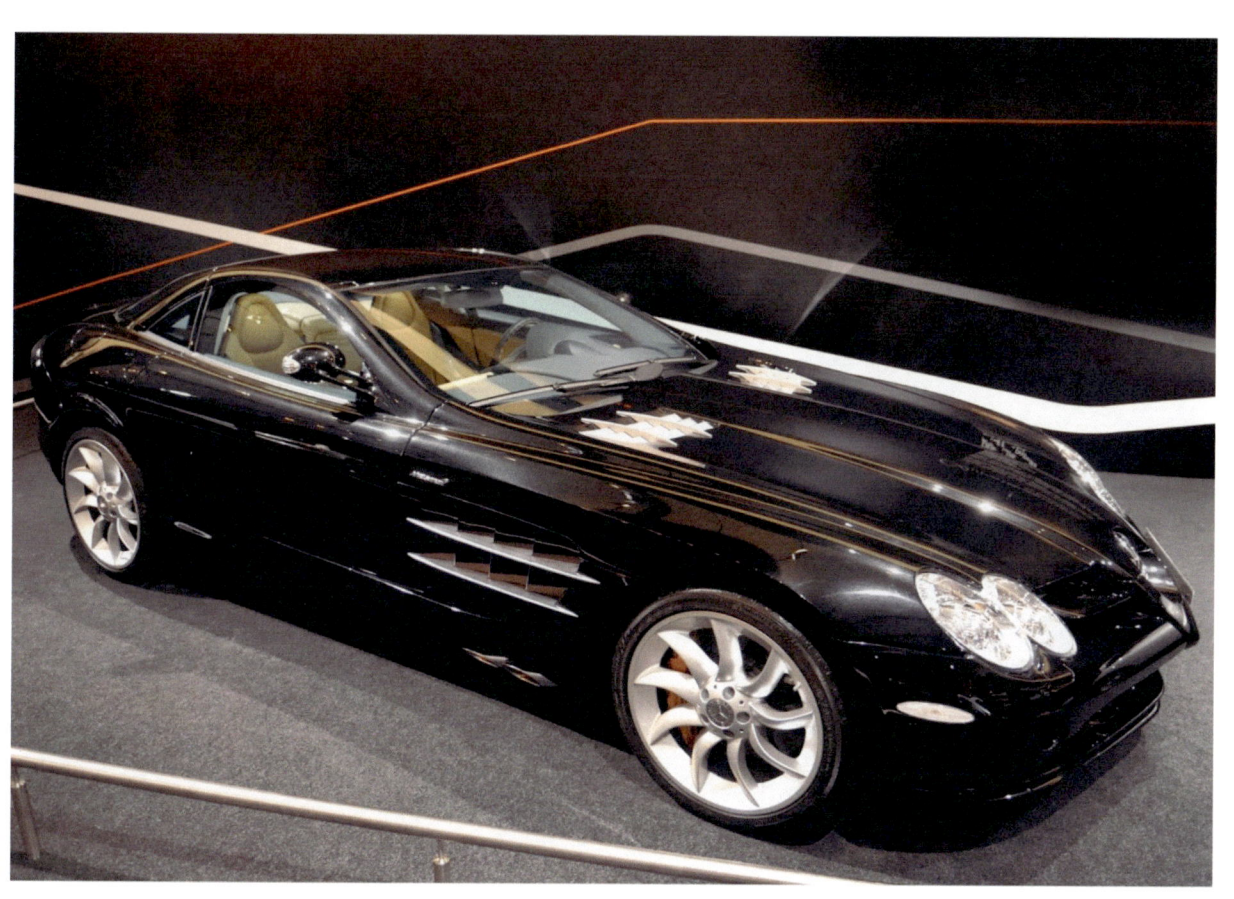

MERCEDES MCLAREN

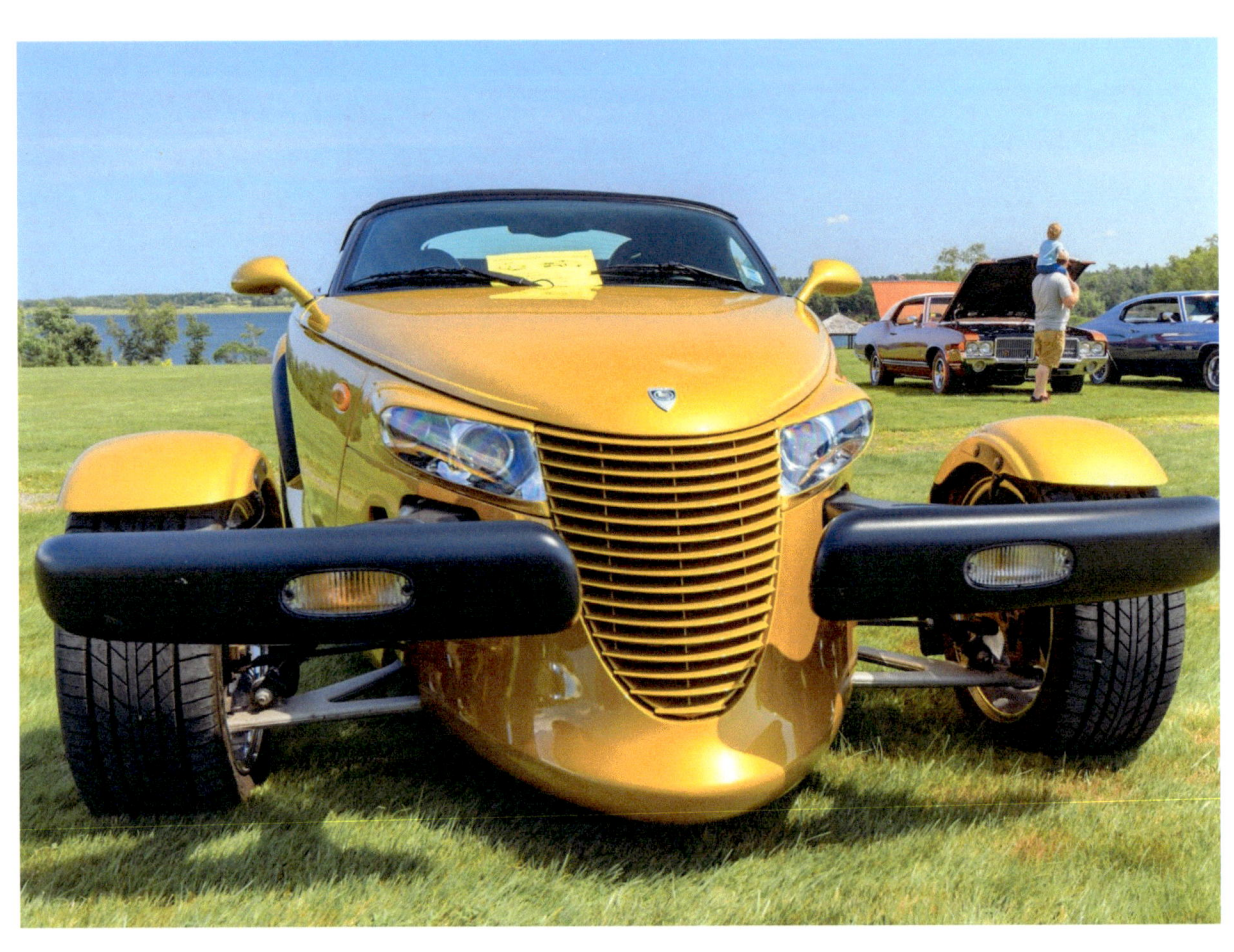

PLYMOUTH PROWLER

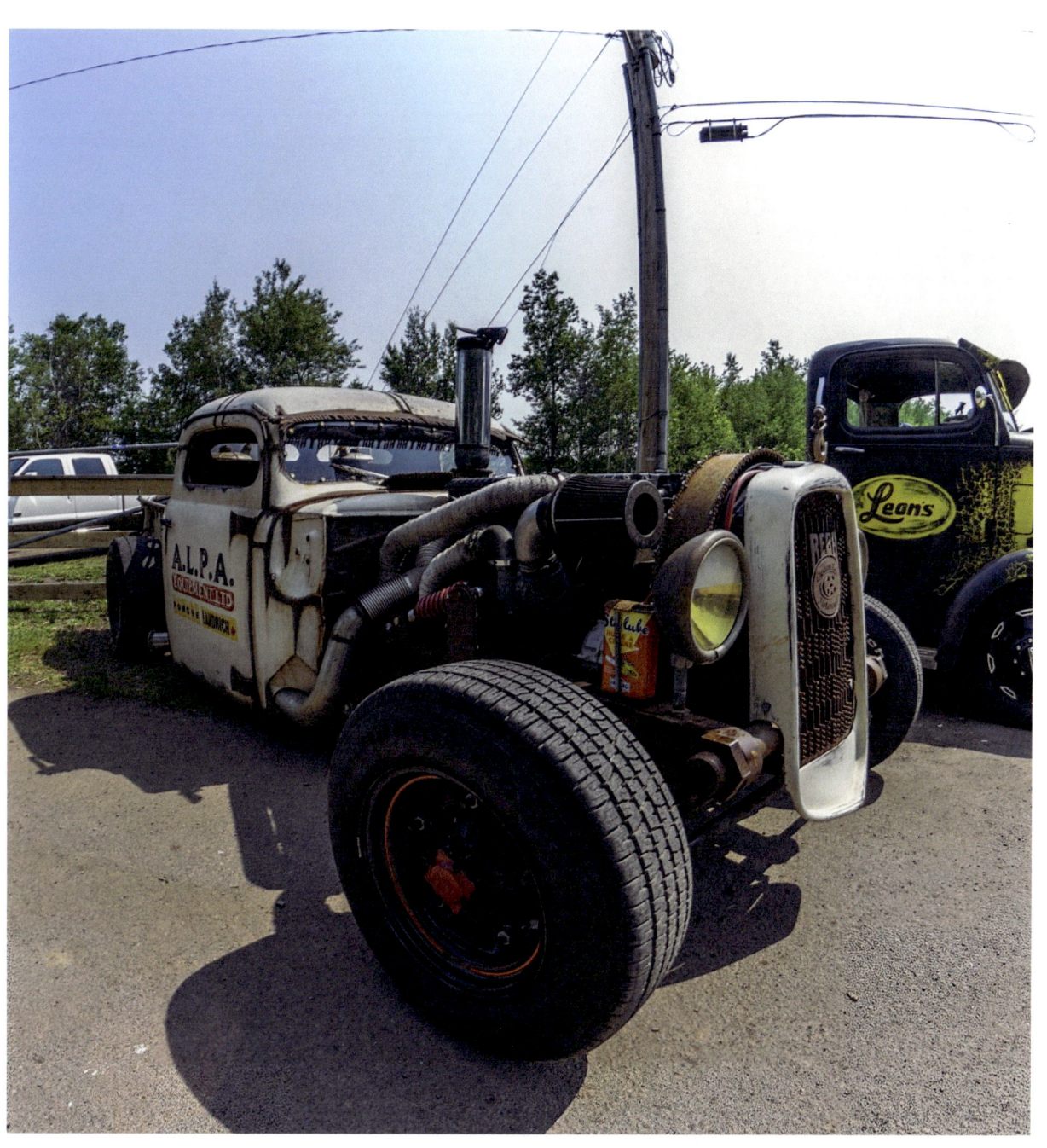

1940 FORD RAT ROD

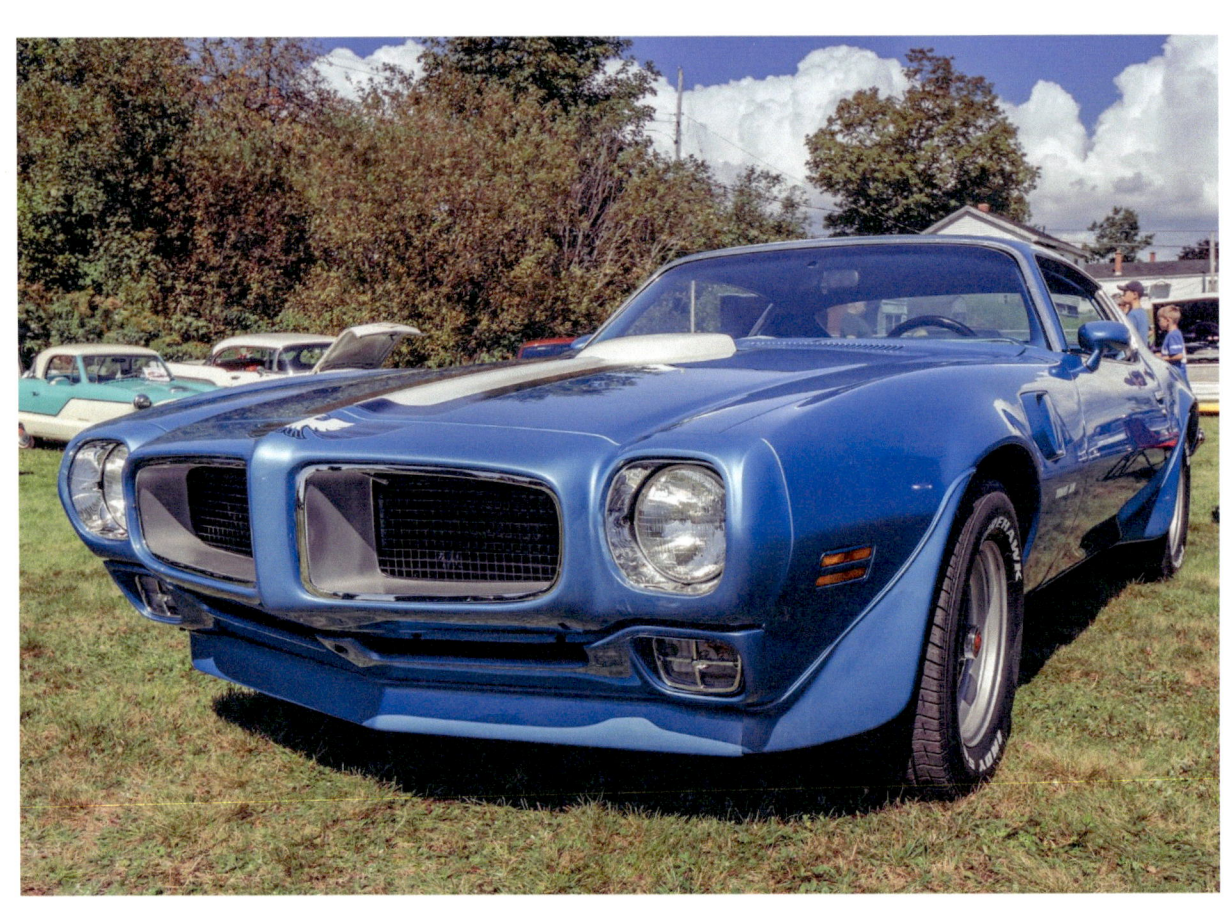

PONTIAC FIREBIRD

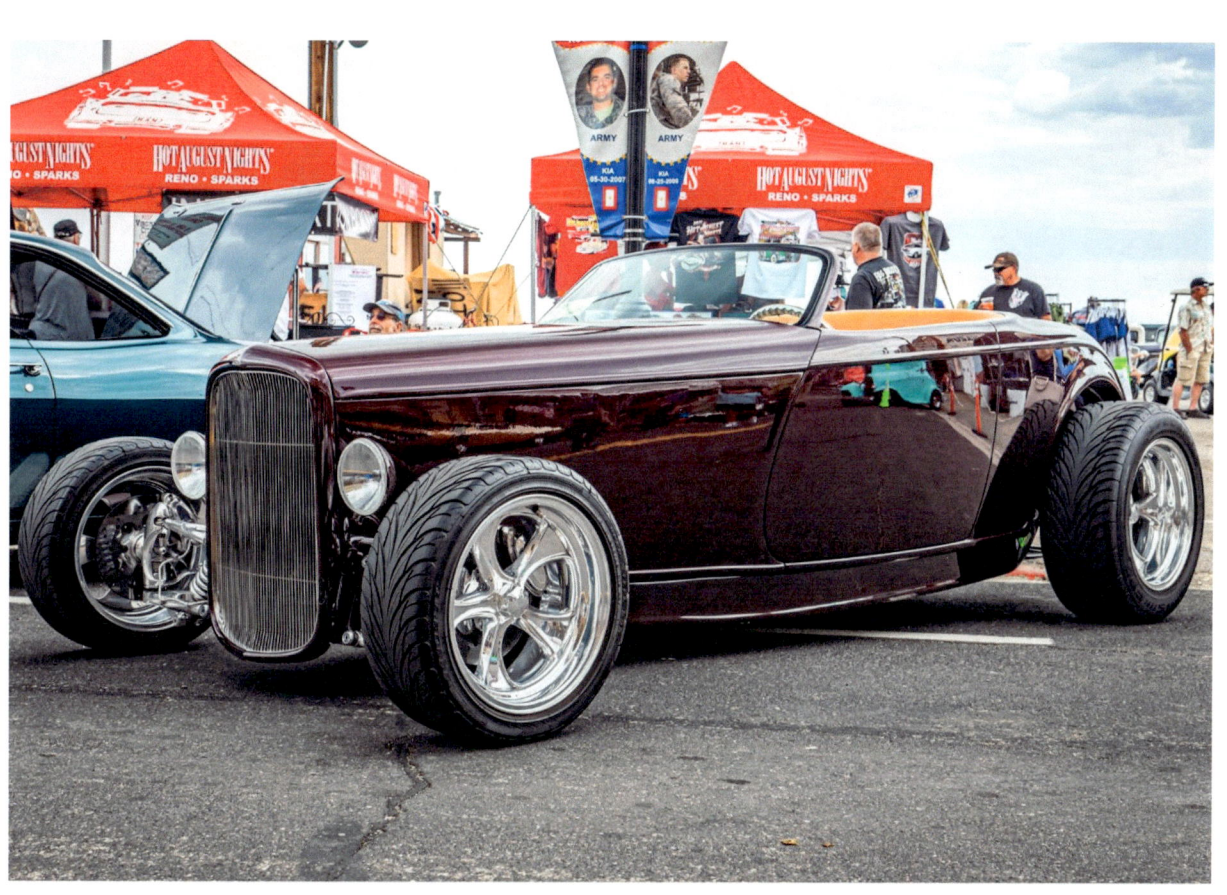

1932 FORD ROADSTER

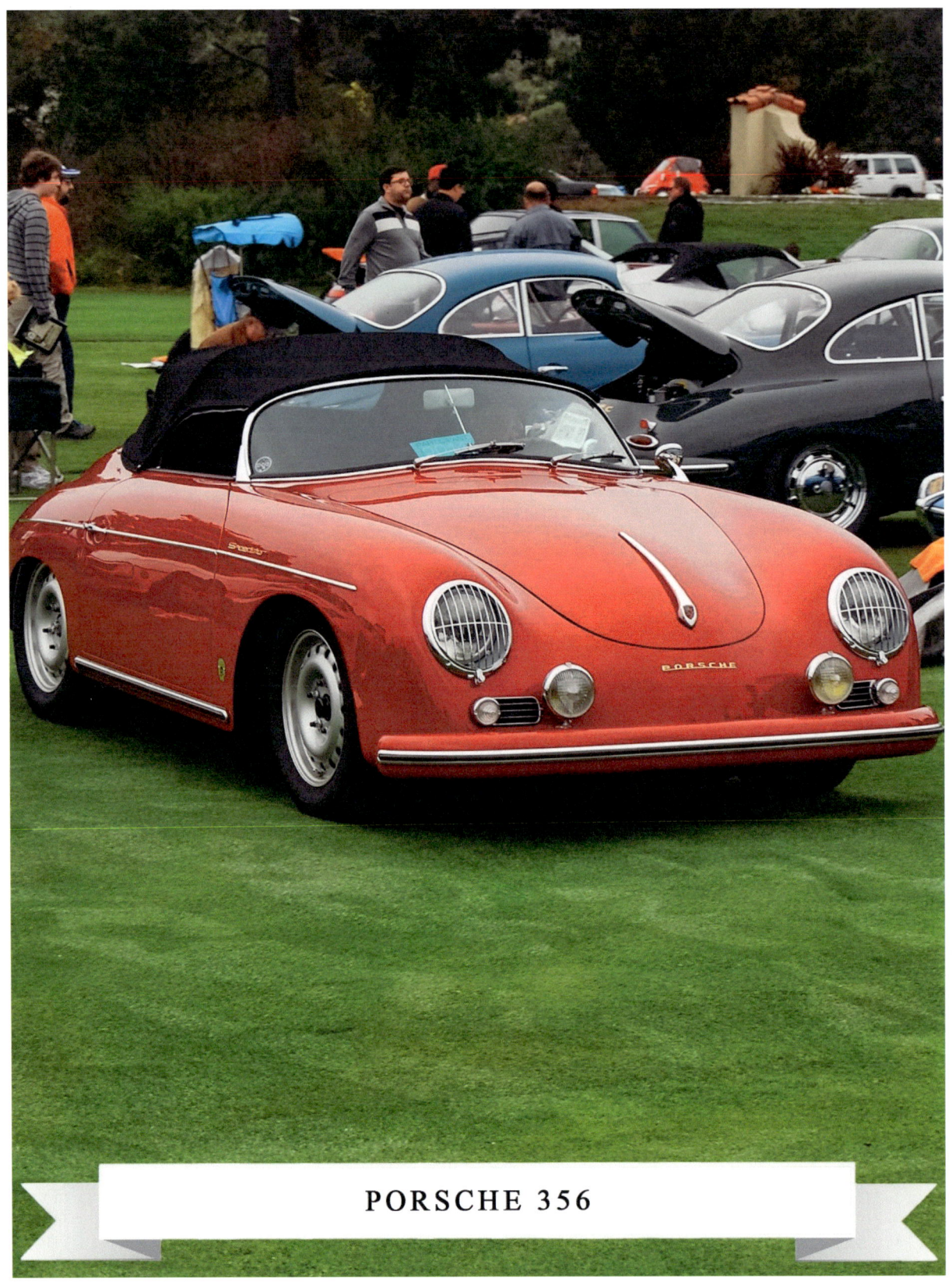

PORSCHE 356

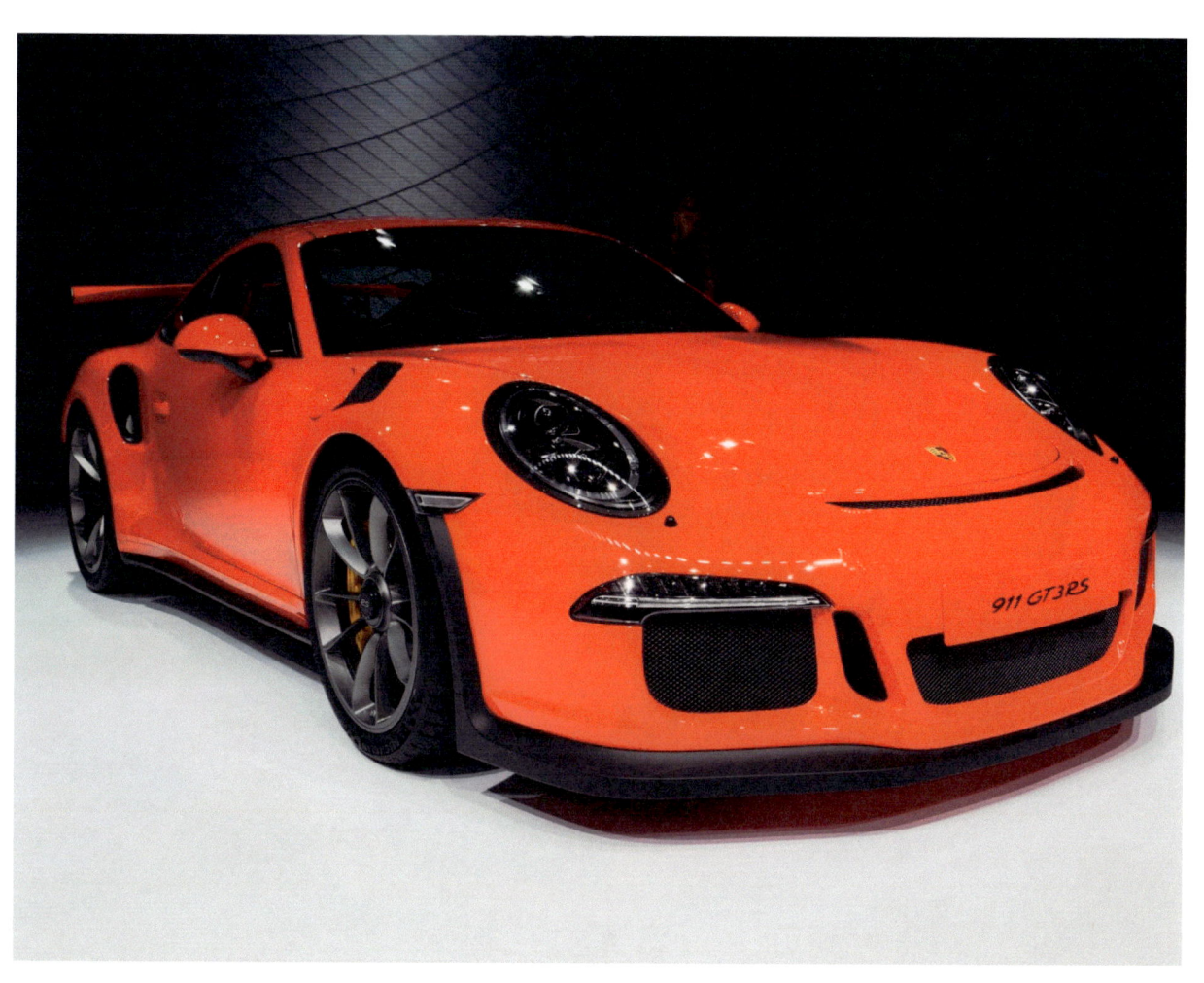

PORSCHE 911

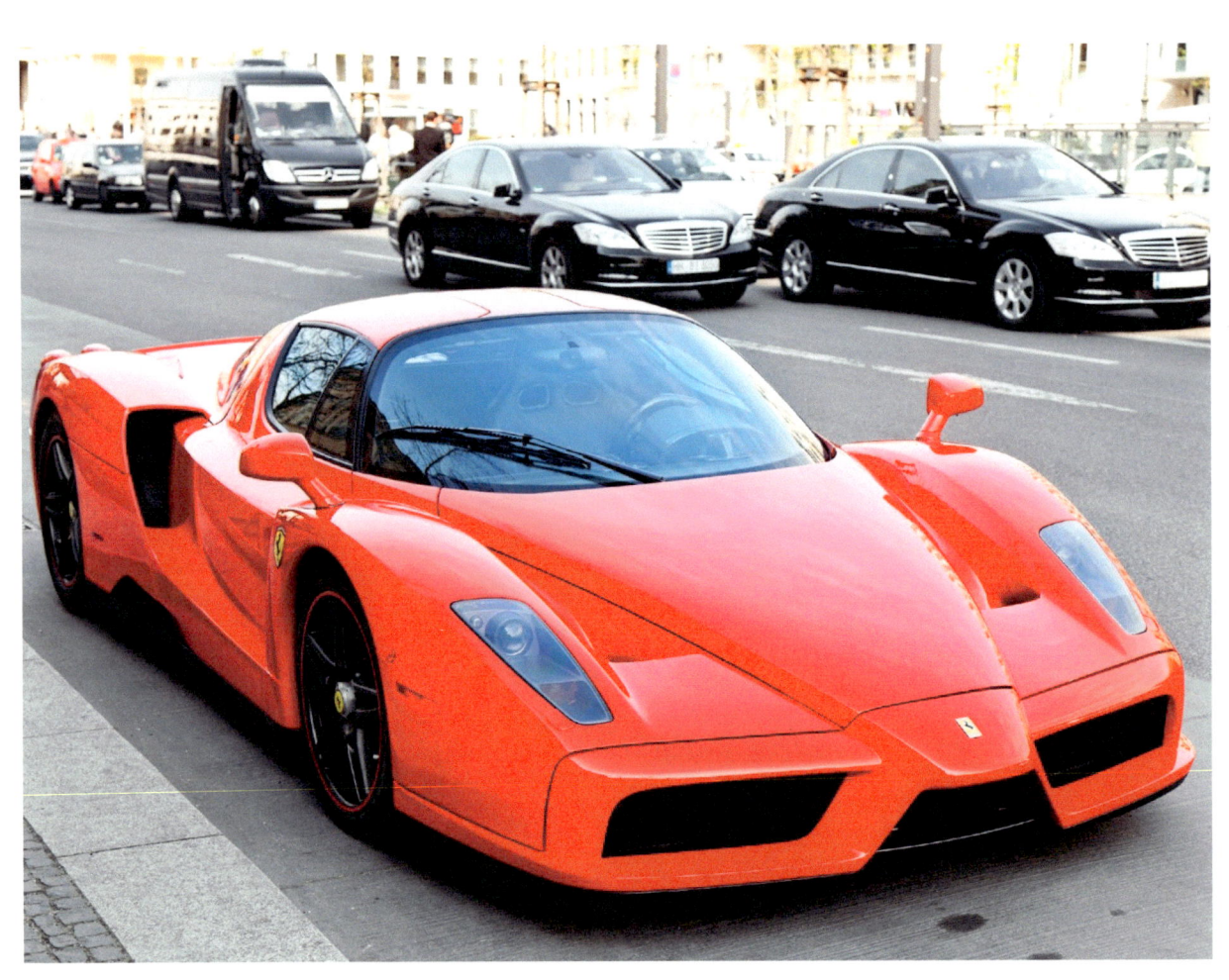

FERRARI ENZO

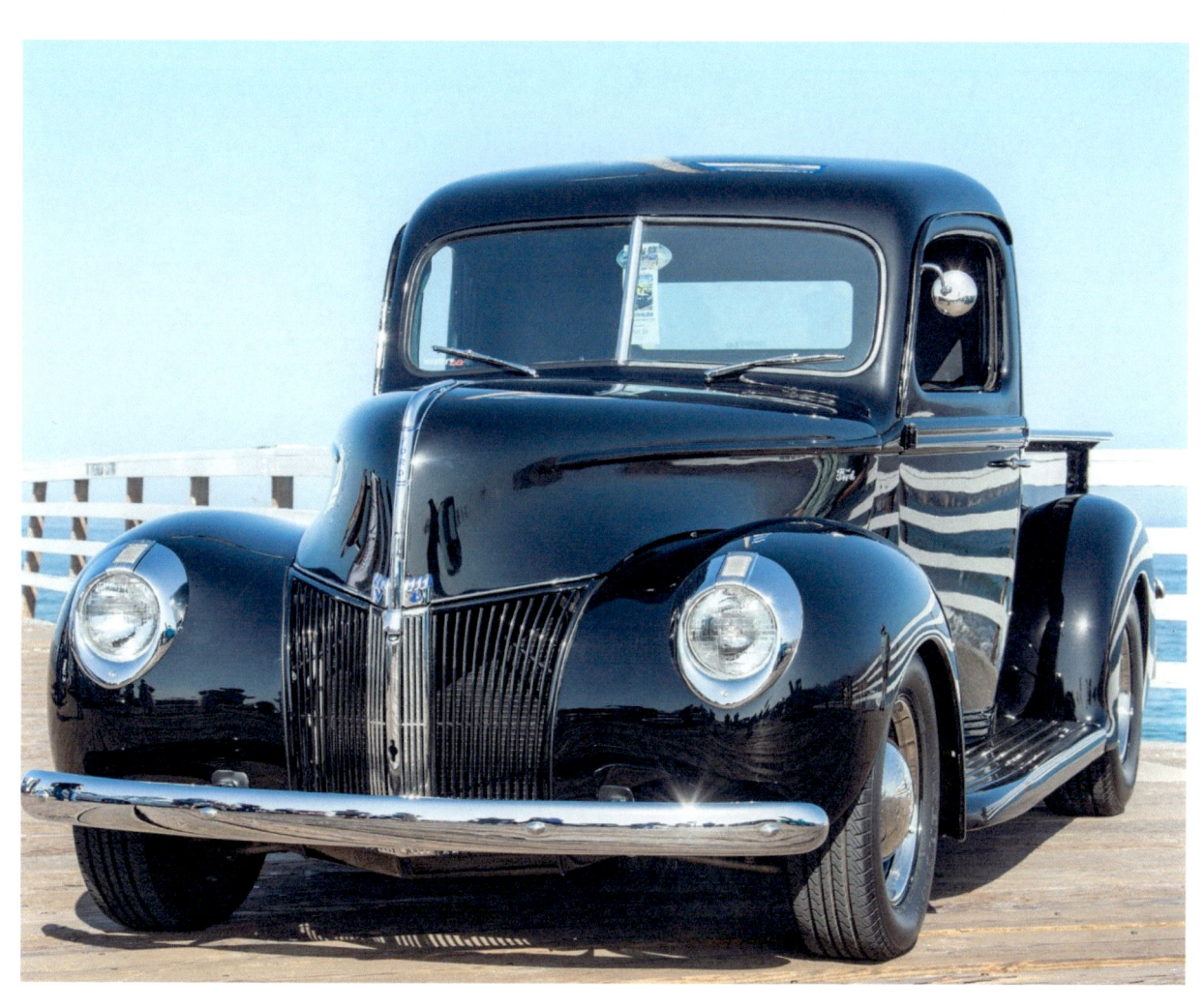

1940 FORD PICKUP

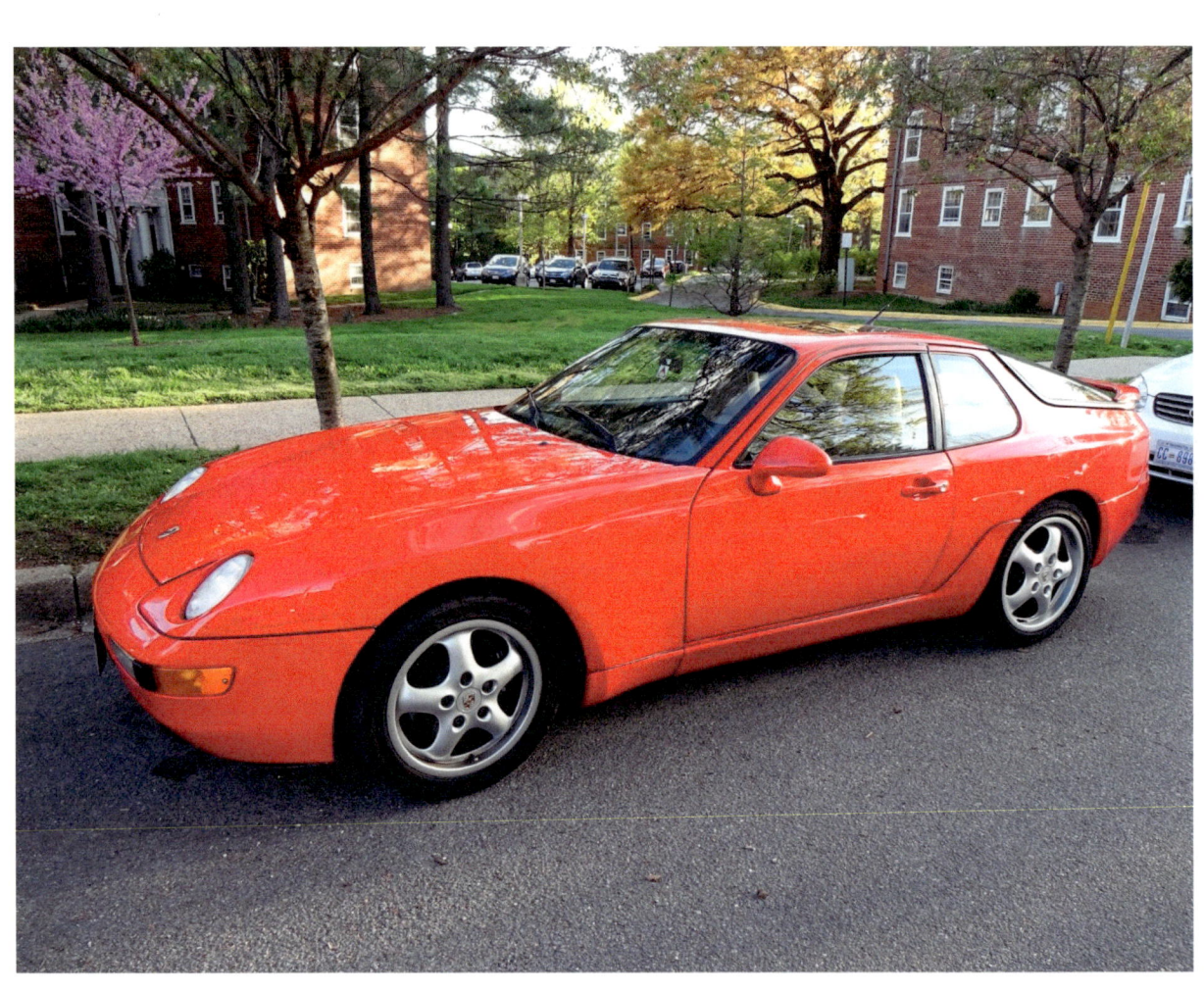

PORSCHE 928

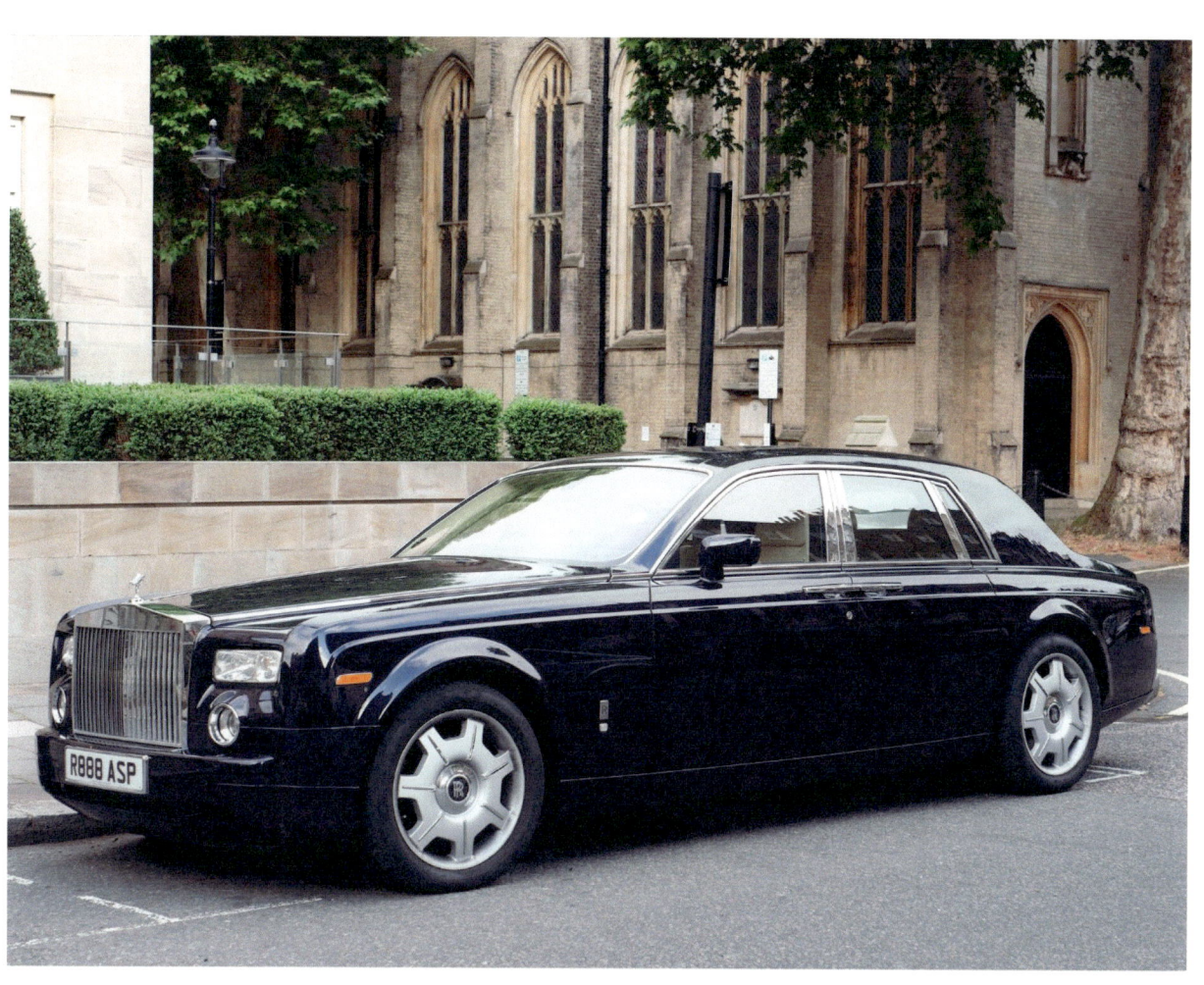

ROLLS ROYCE PHANTOM

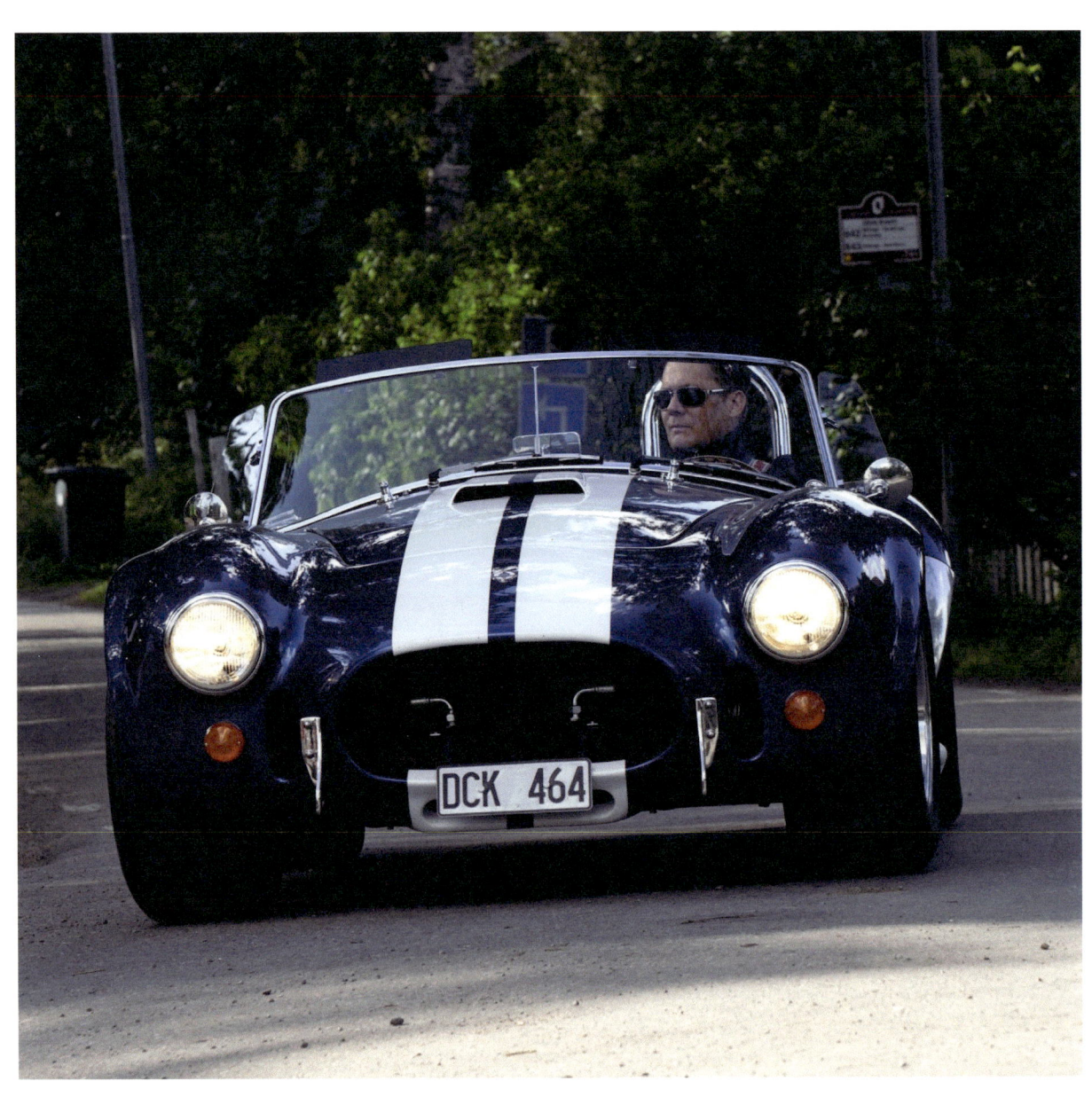

SHELBY COBRA

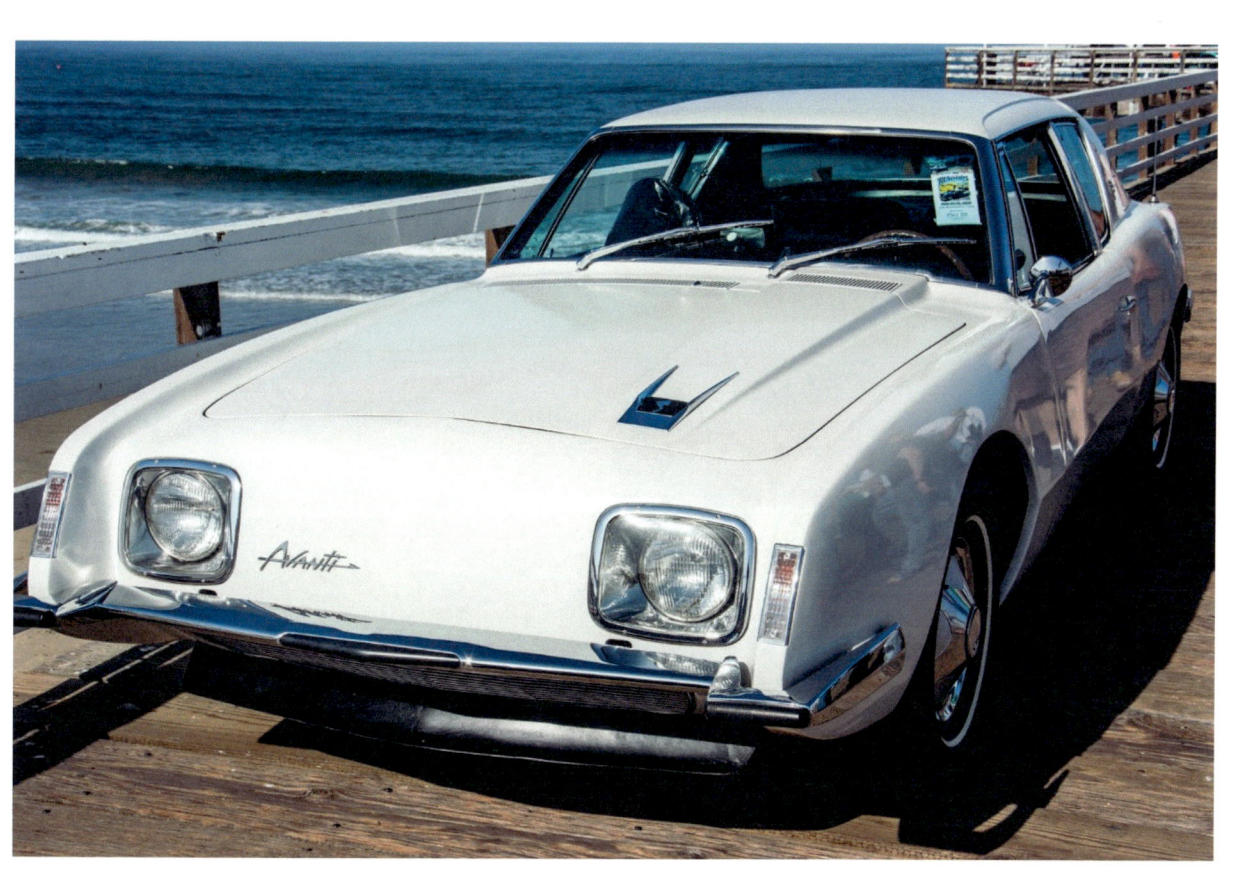

STUDEBAKER AVANTI

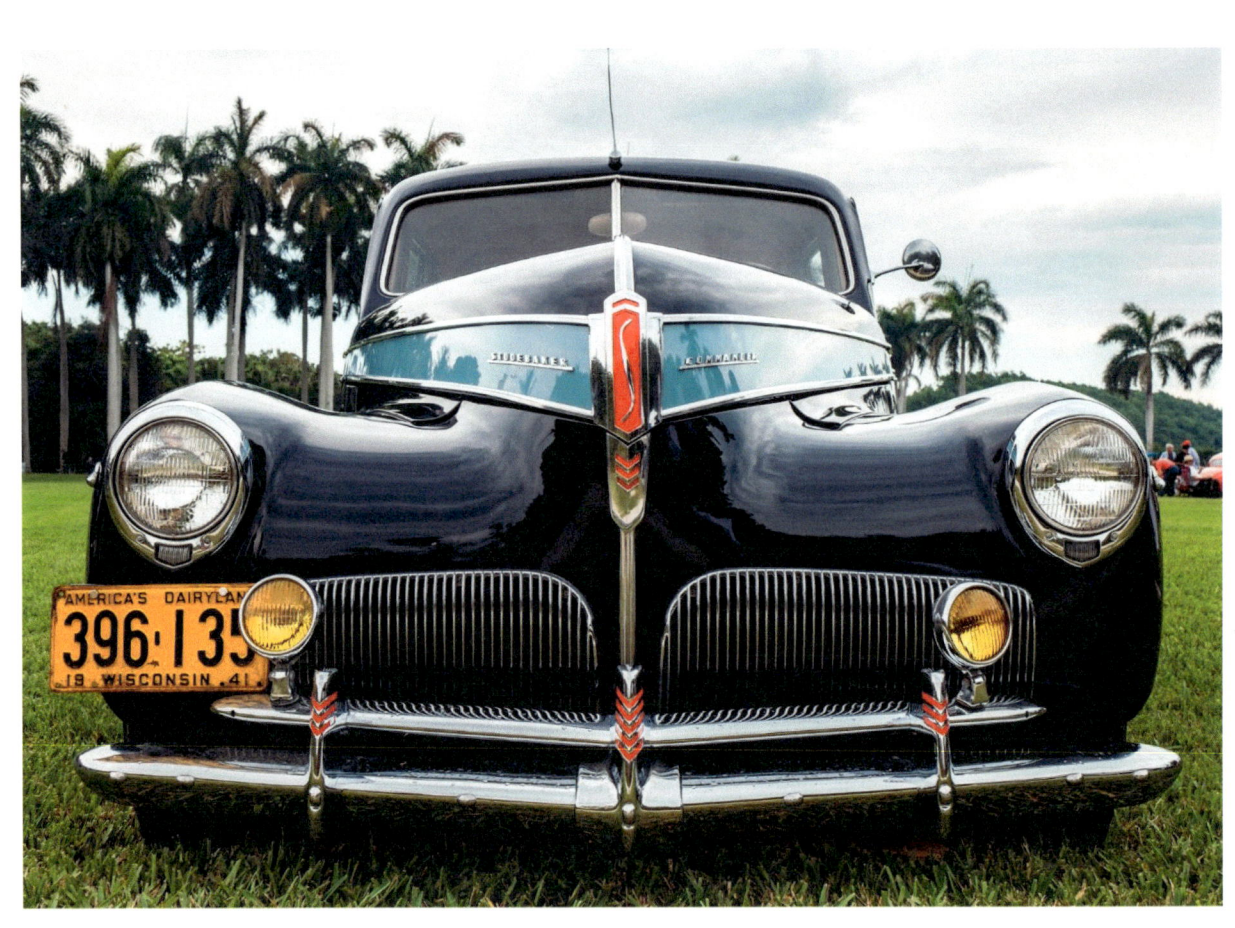

STUDEBAKER COMMANDER

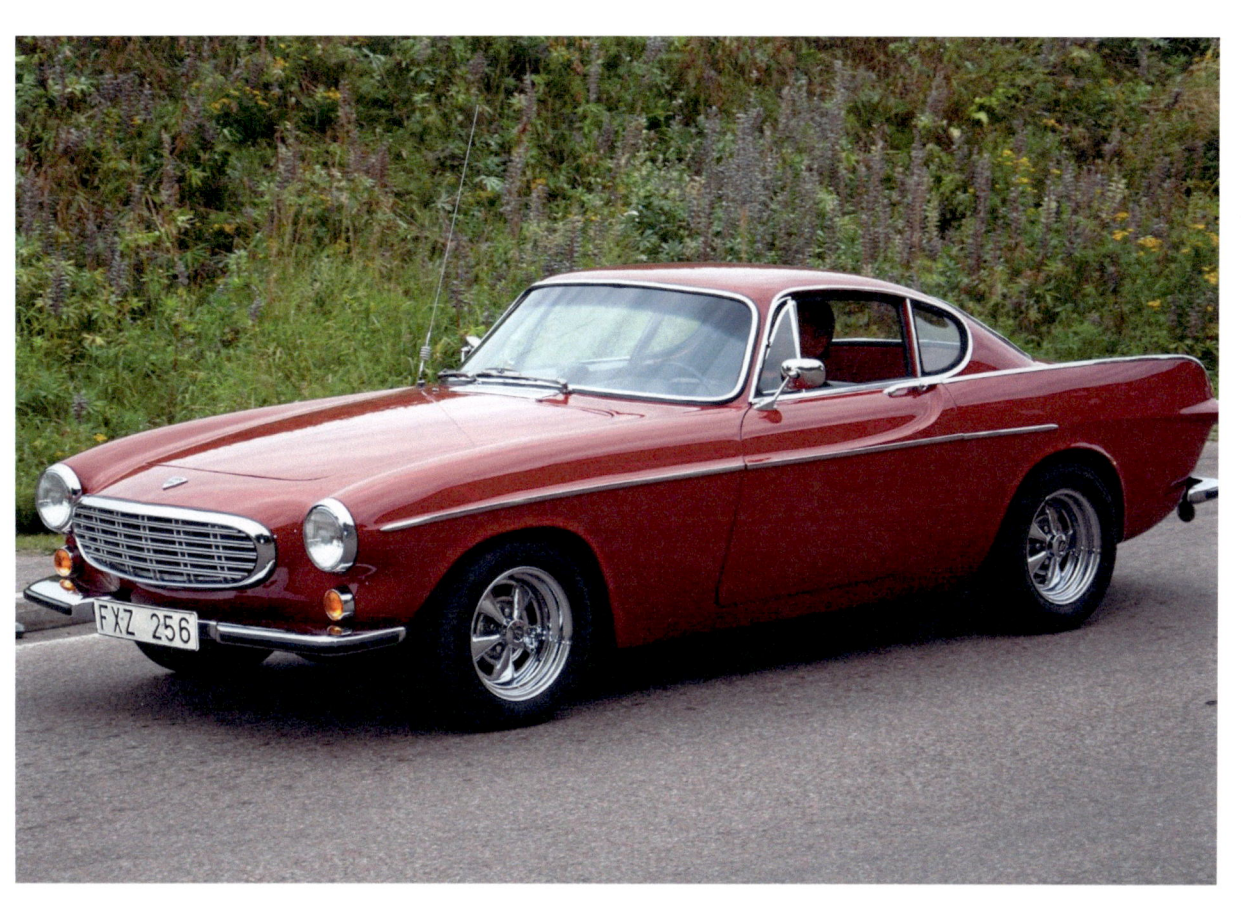

VOLVO P1800

Thank you

Thanks for your interest in our books.

Please consider purchasing our other books available now at Amazon.com.

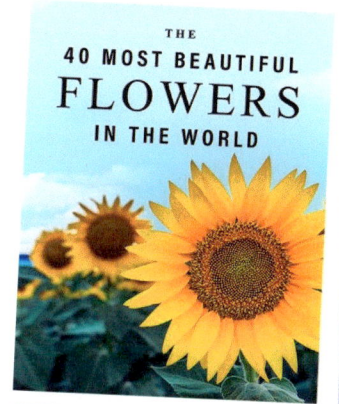
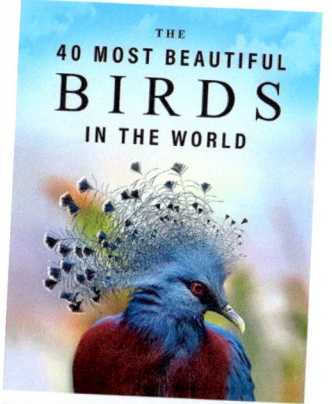
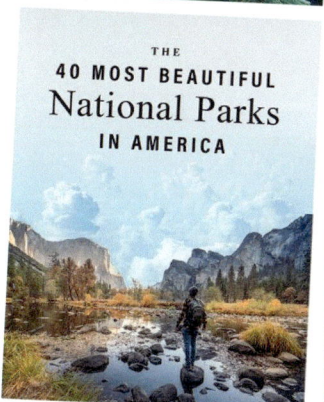
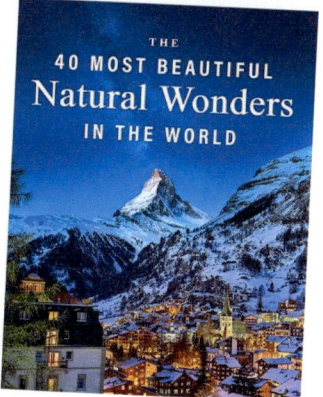

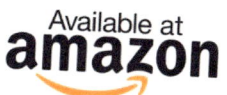

(Just search for "Blue Clover Books" on Amazon.)

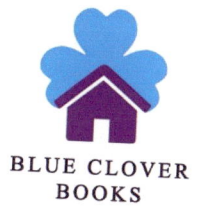

Made in United States
Troutdale, OR
09/15/2024